101 FACE CHARTS

ISBN-13: 978-1979493468

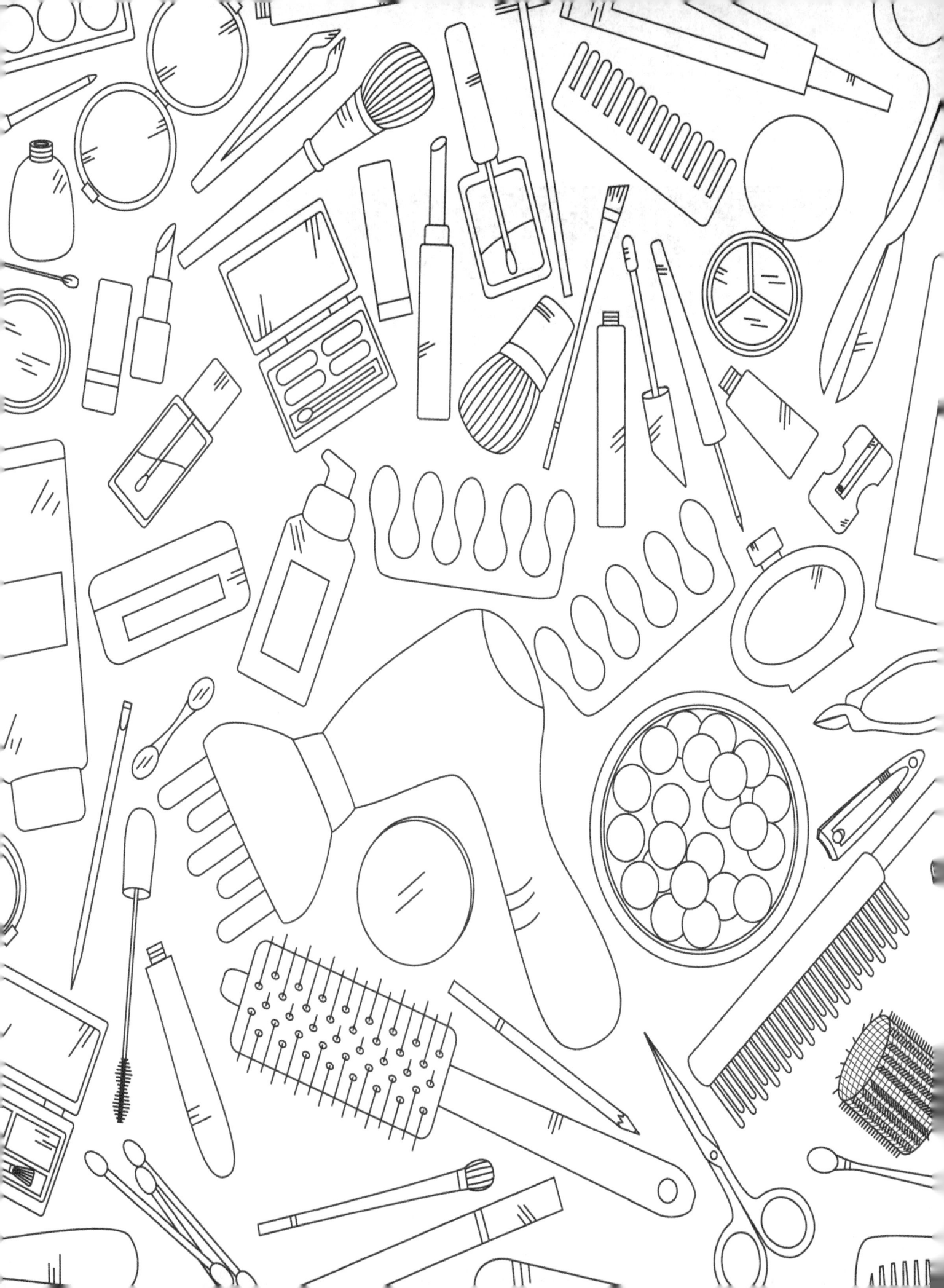

Contents

Client Name / Reference Number	Page

Contents

Client Name / Reference Number	Page

Contents

Client Name / Reference Number	Page

Contents

Client Name / Reference Number	Page

Contents

Client Name / Reference Number	Page

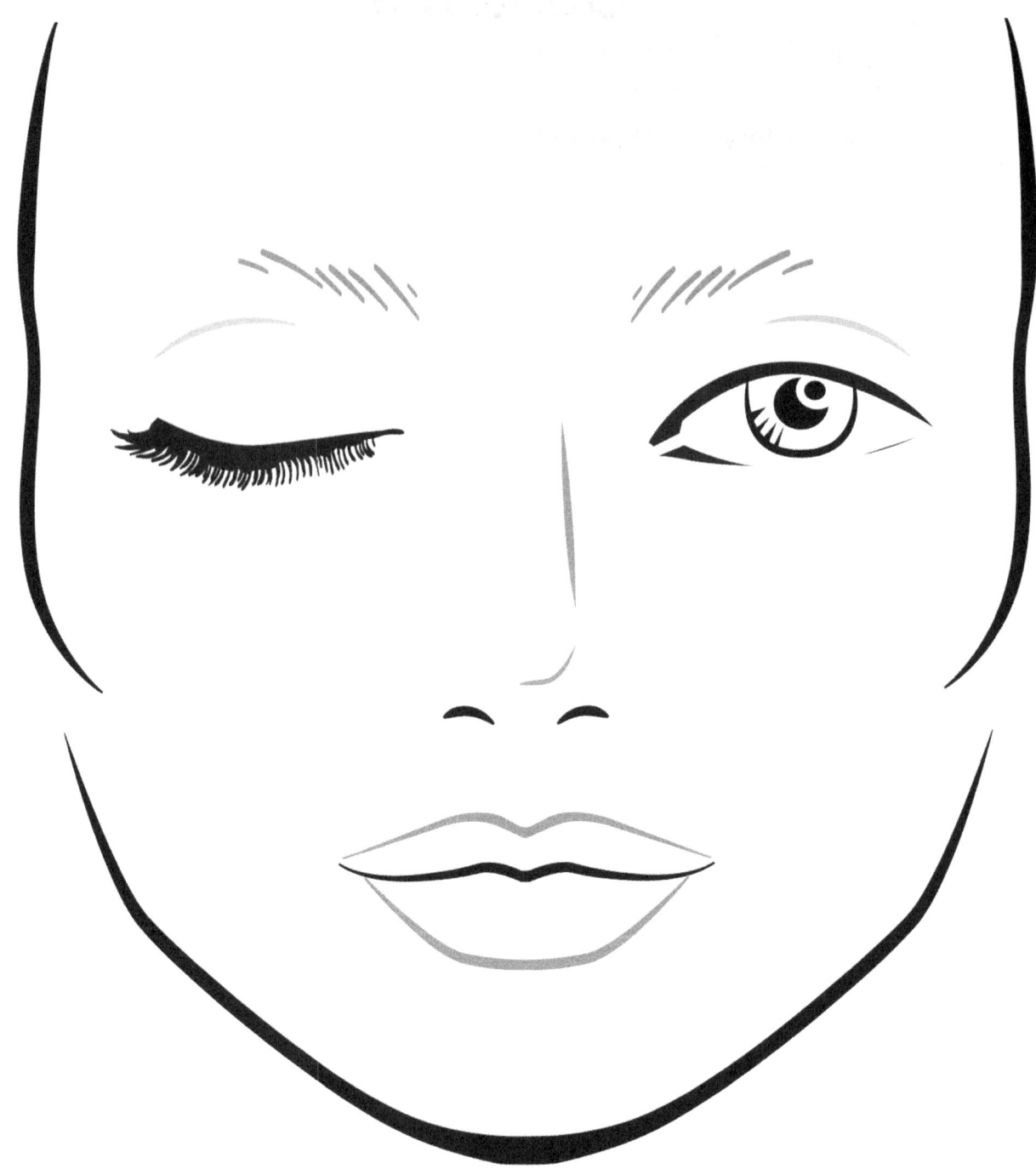

Skin	Eyes	Lips

Client Name: ....
Phone Number: ....
Email Address: ....
Makeup Look: Daytime / Evening / Wedding / Party / Other / (Circle as appropriate).

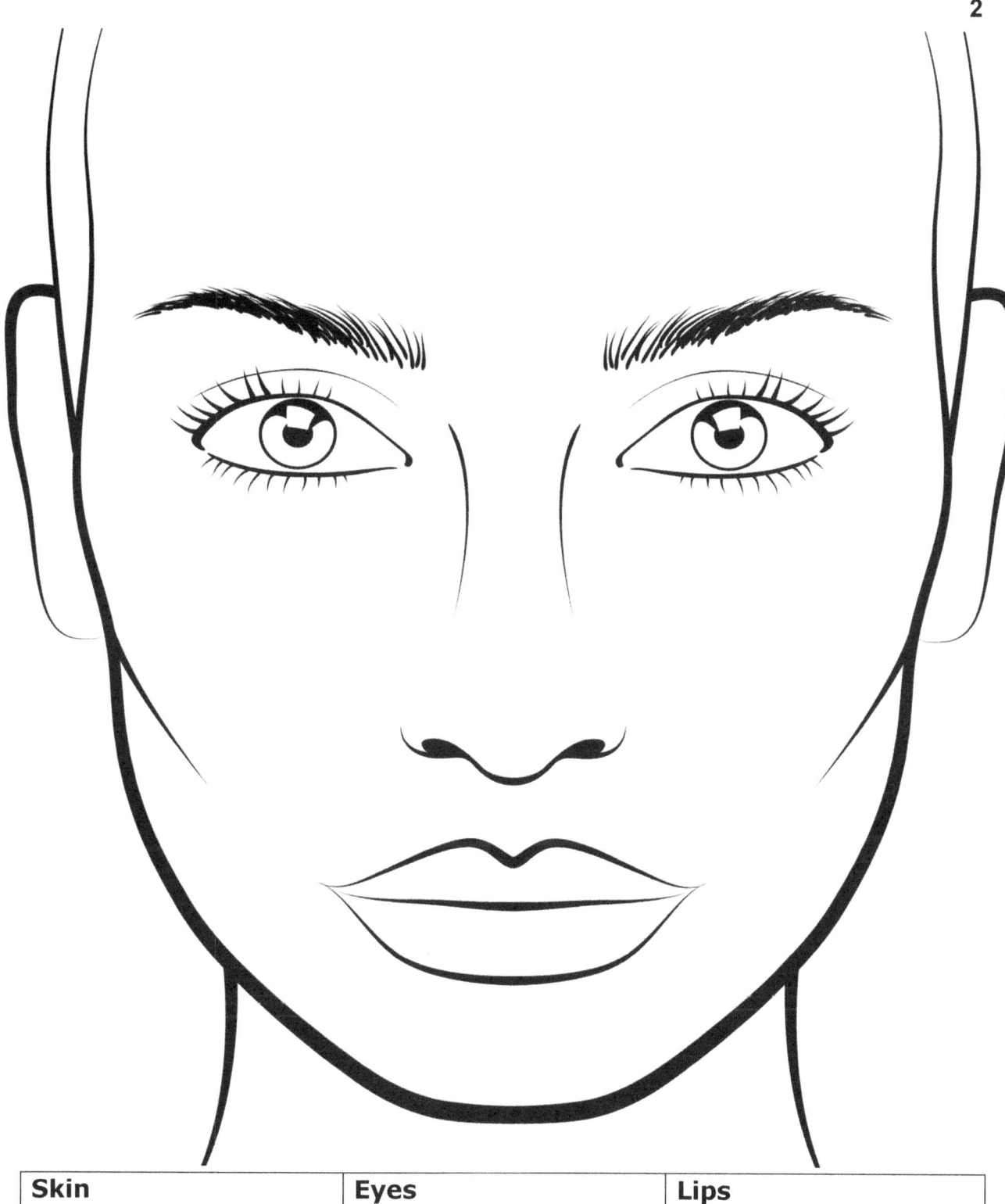

Skin	Eyes	Lips

Client Name: ....
Phone Number: ....
Email Address: ....
Makeup Look: Daytime / Evening / Wedding / Party / Other / (Circle as appropriate).

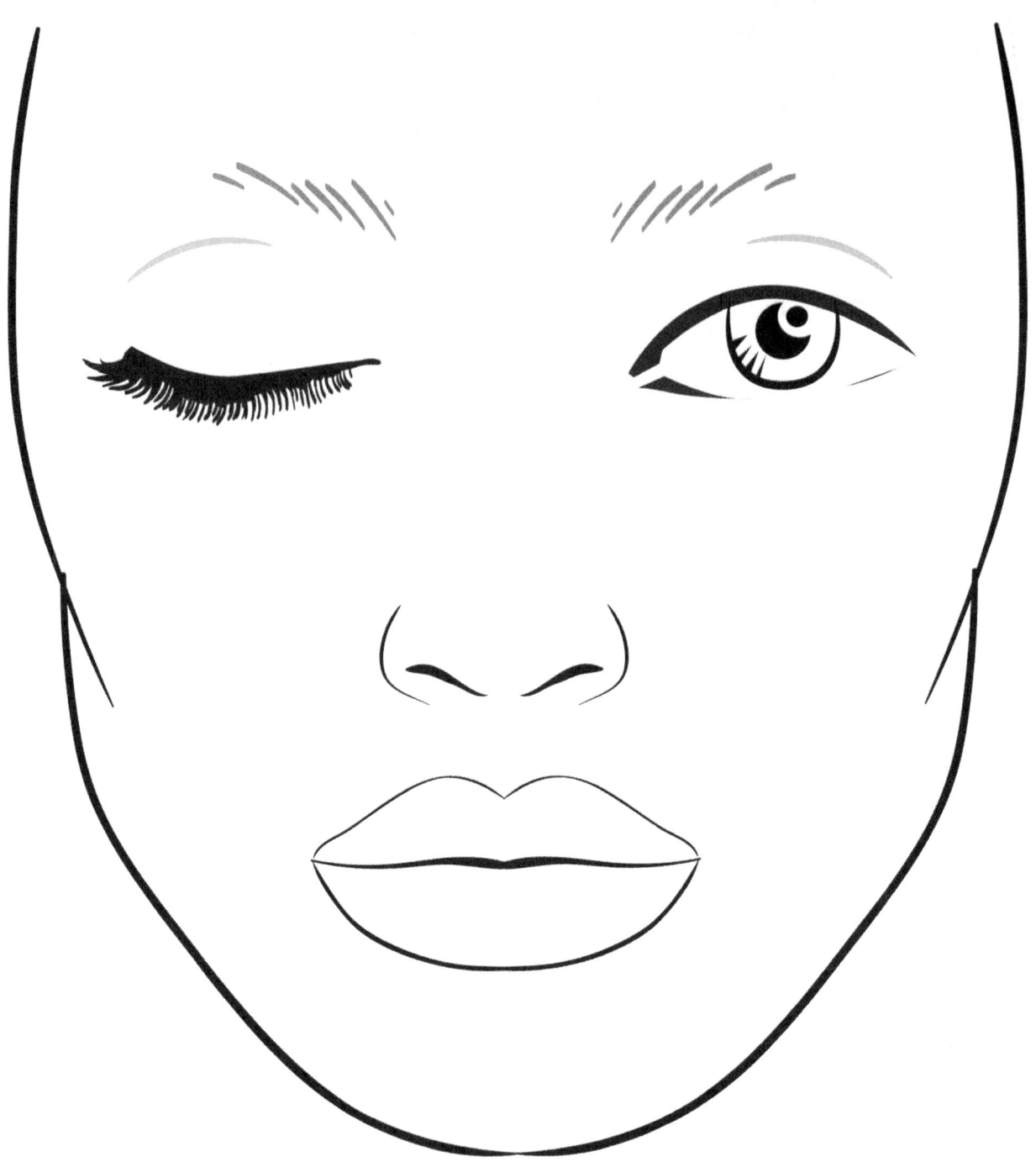

Skin	Eyes	Lips

Client Name: ....
Phone Number: ....
Email Address: ....
Makeup Look: Daytime / Evening / Wedding / Party / Other / (Circle as appropriate).

Skin	Eyes	Lips

Client Name: ....
Phone Number: ....
Email Address: ....
Makeup Look: Daytime / Evening / Wedding / Party / Other / (Circle as appropriate).

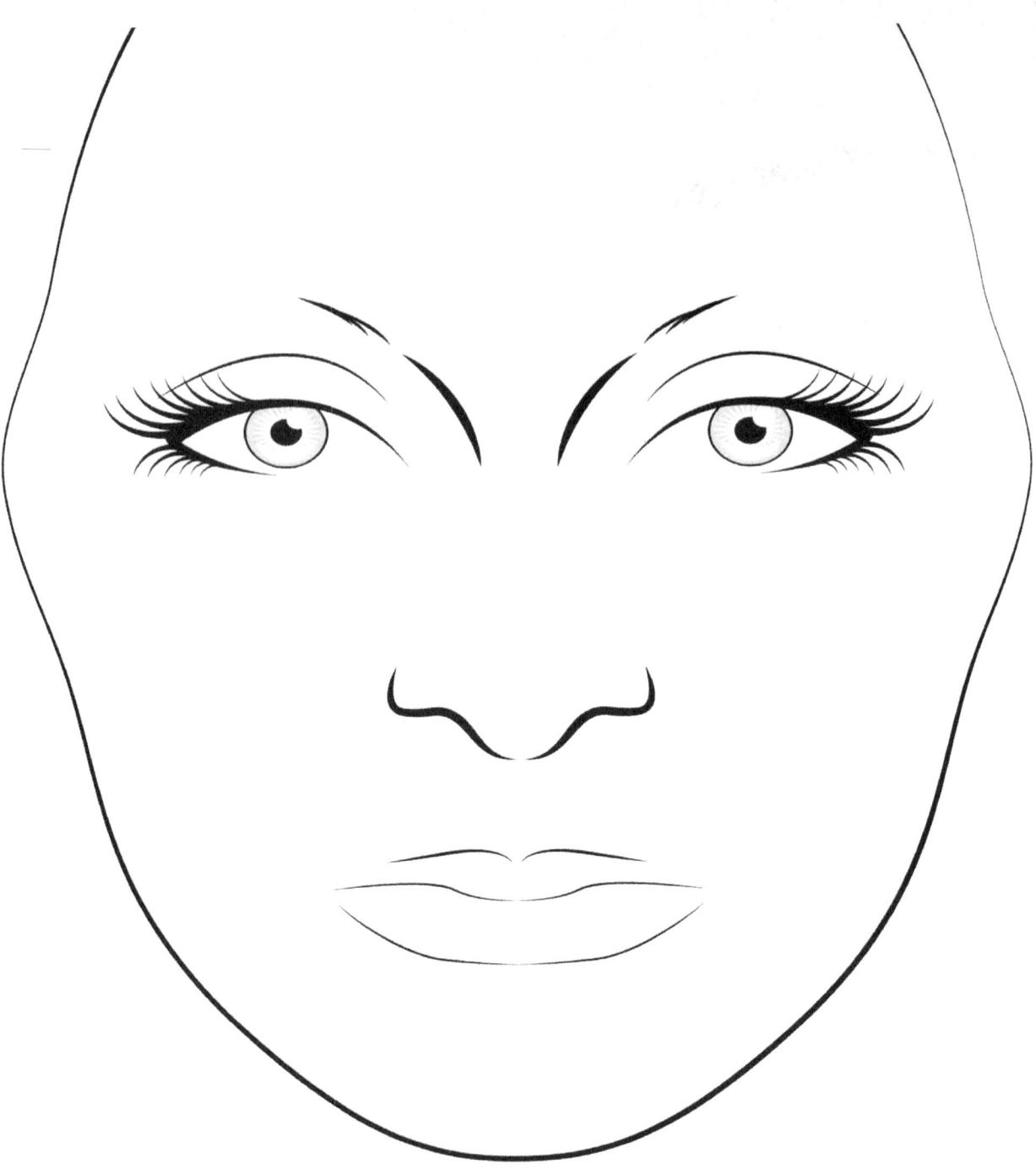

Skin	Eyes	Lips

Client Name: ....
Phone Number: ....
Email Address: ....
Makeup Look: Daytime / Evening / Wedding / Party / Other / (Circle as appropriate).

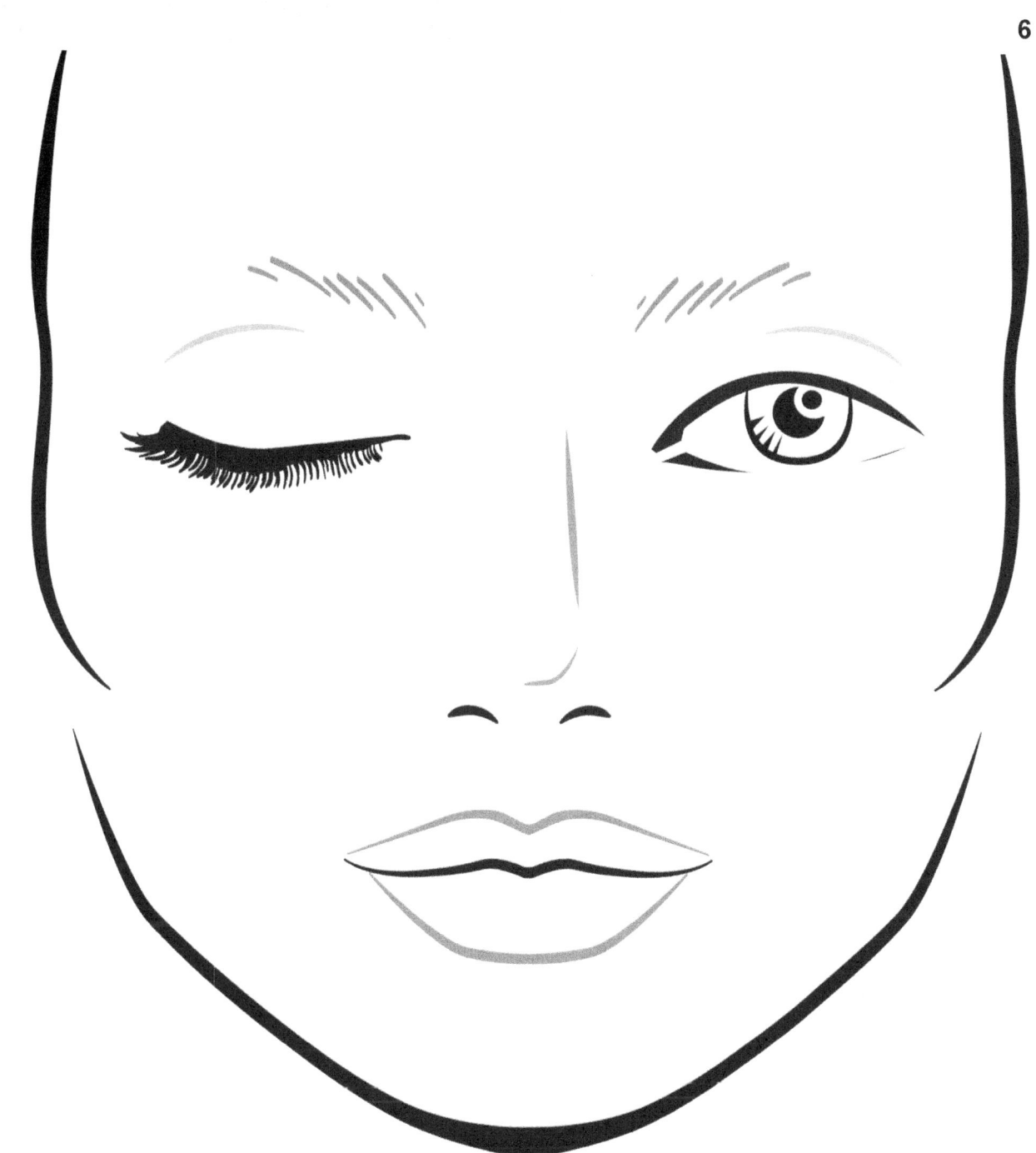

Skin	Eyes	Lips

Client Name: ....
Phone Number: ....
Email Address: ....
Makeup Look: Daytime / Evening / Wedding / Party / Other / (Circle as appropriate).

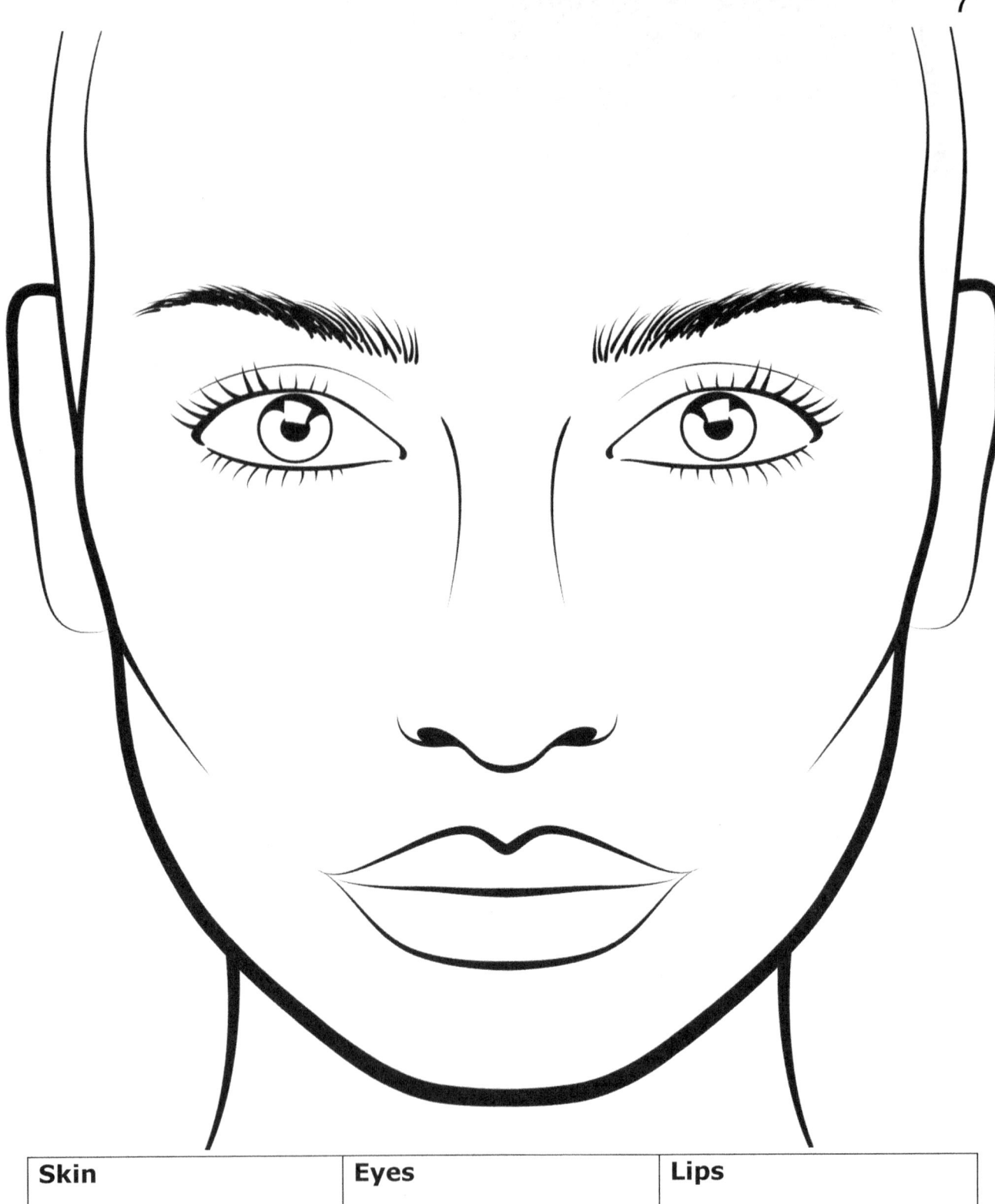

Skin	Eyes	Lips

Client Name: ....

Phone Number: ....

Email Address: ....

Makeup Look: Daytime / Evening / Wedding / Party / Other / (Circle as appropriate).

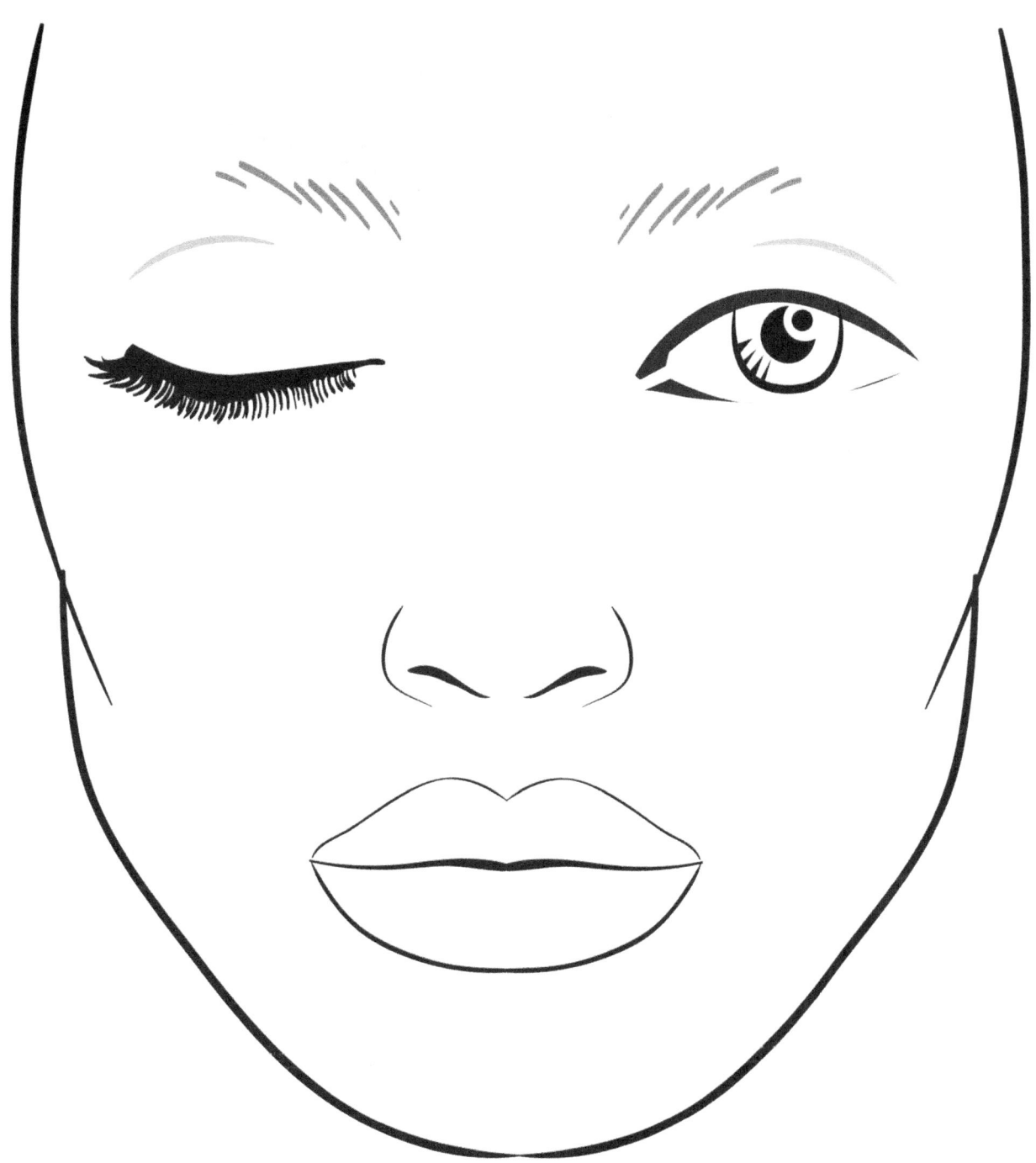

Skin	Eyes	Lips

Client Name: ....
Phone Number: ....
Email Address: ....
Makeup Look: Daytime / Evening / Wedding / Party / Other / (Circle as appropriate).

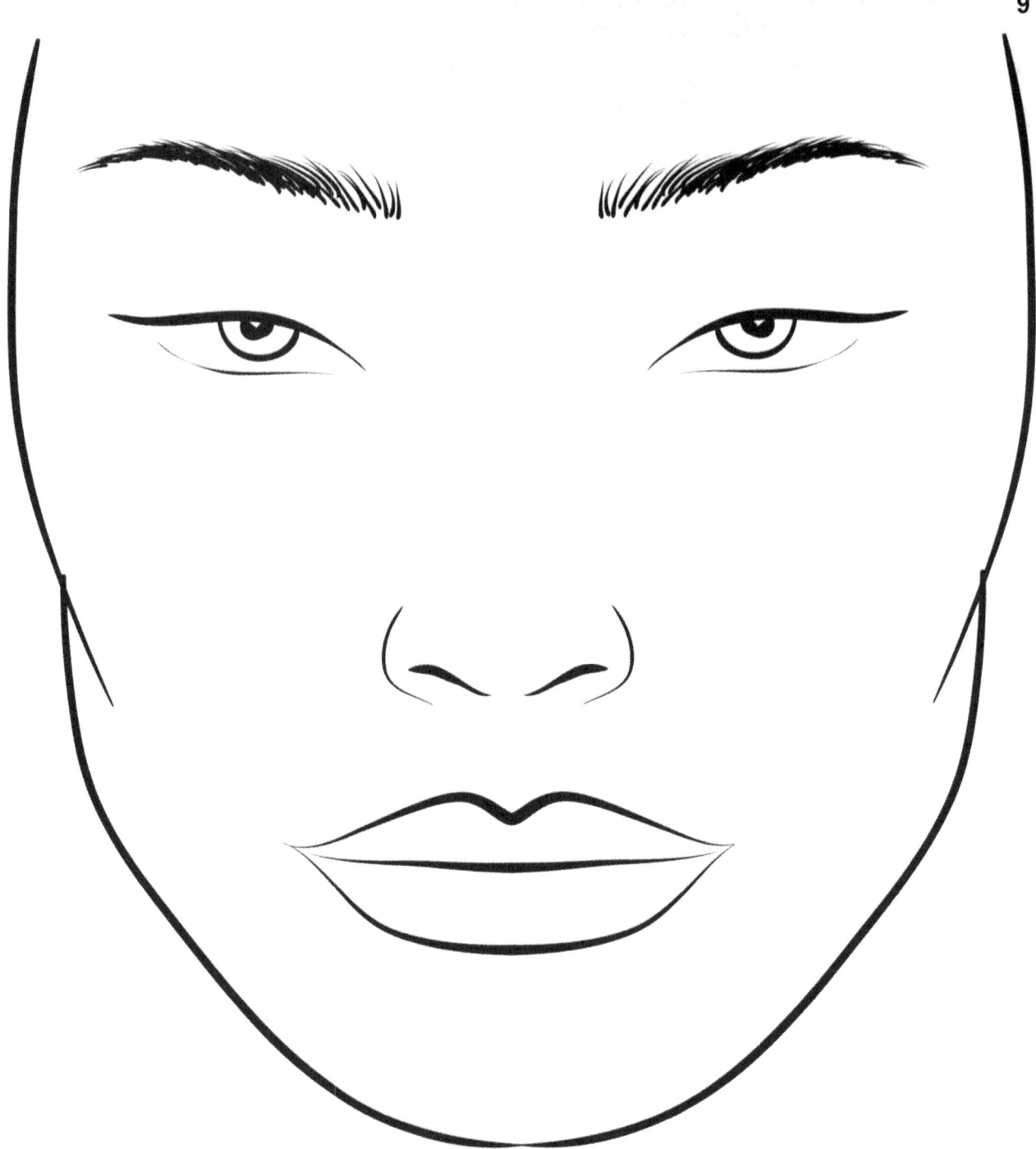

Skin	Eyes	Lips

Client Name: ....
Phone Number: ....
Email Address: ....
Makeup Look: Daytime / Evening / Wedding / Party / Other / (Circle as appropriate).

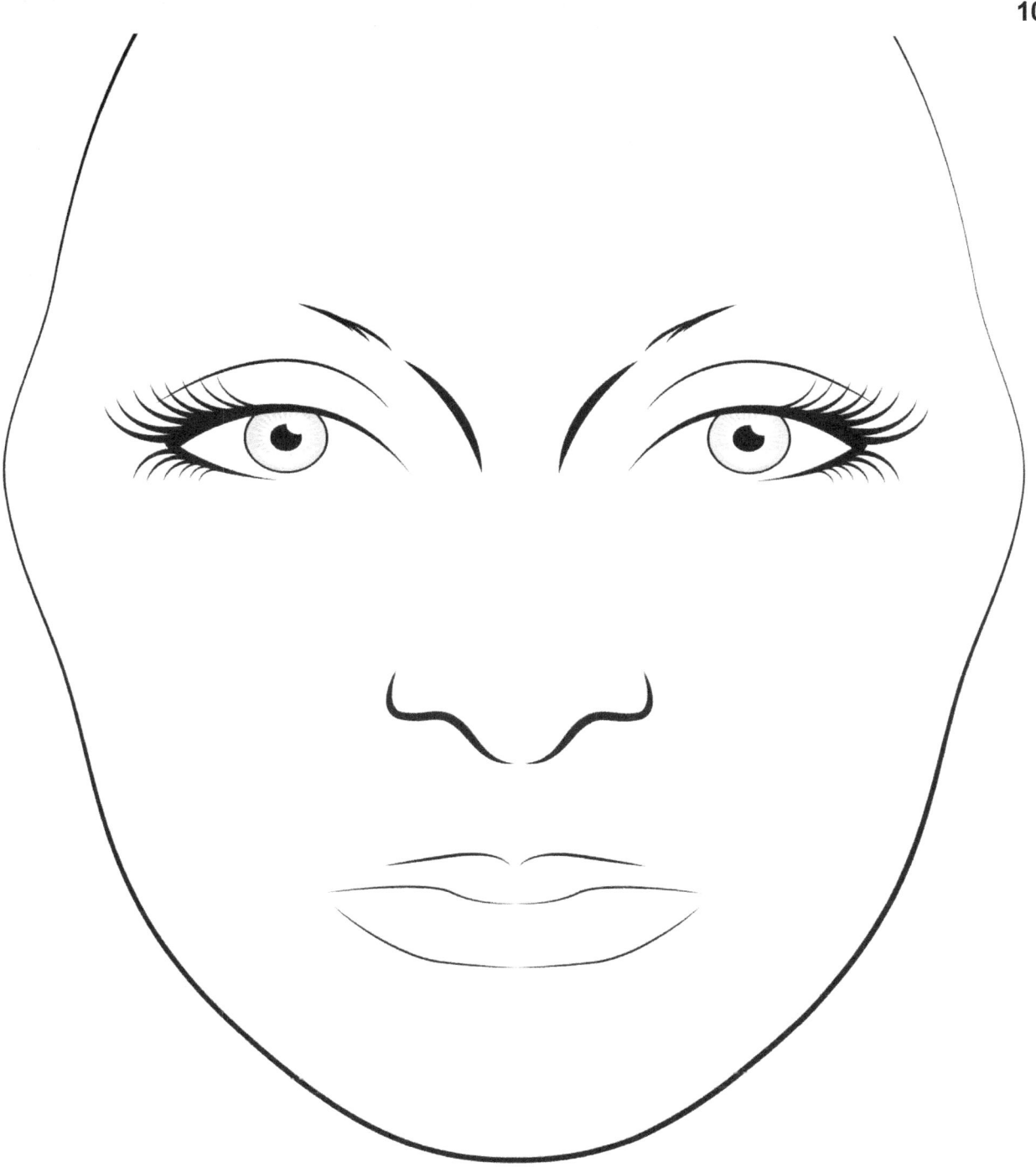

Skin	Eyes	Lips

Client Name: ....
Phone Number: ....
Email Address: ....
Makeup Look: Daytime / Evening / Wedding / Party / Other / (Circle as appropriate).

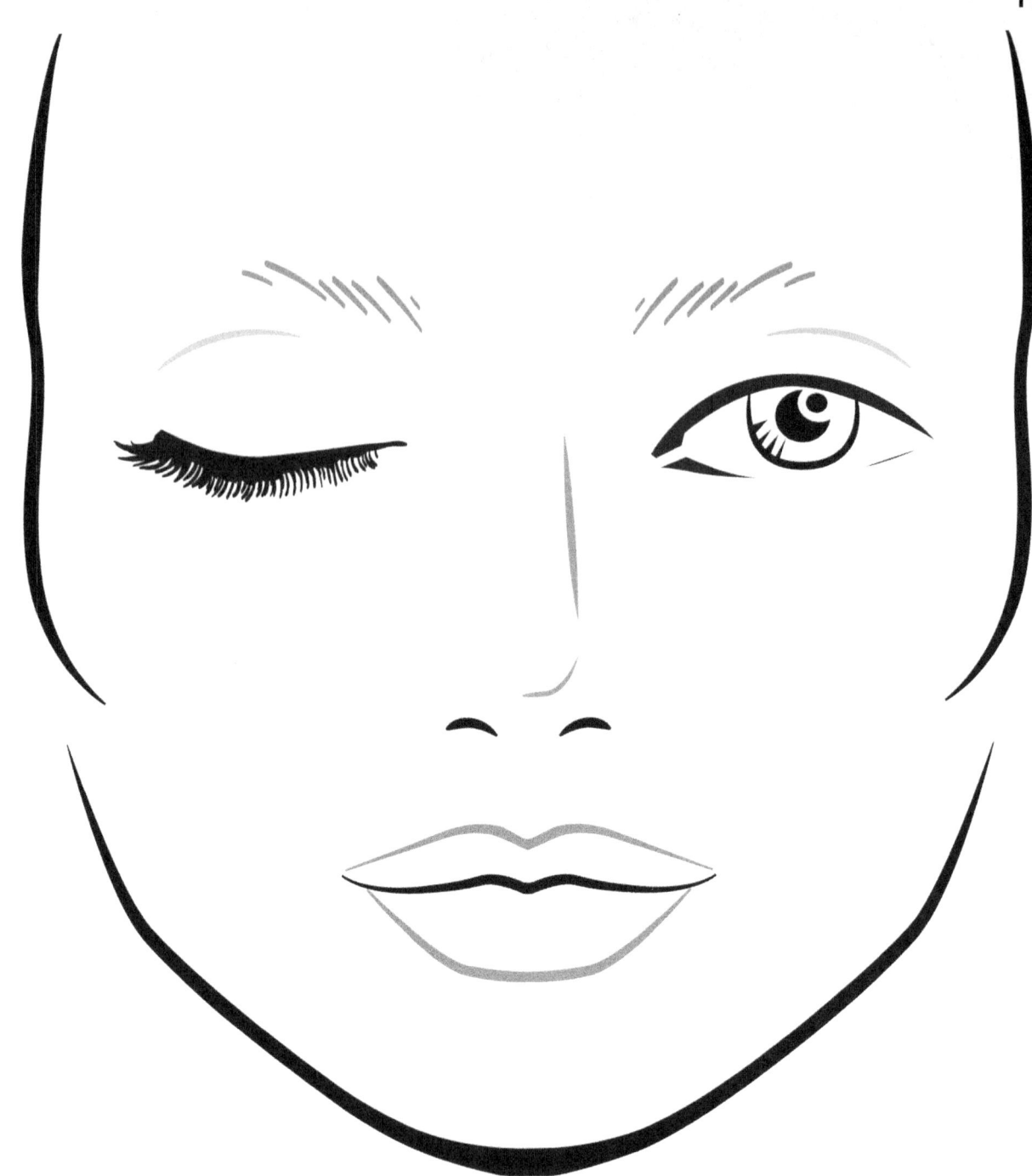

Skin	Eyes	Lips

Client Name: ....
Phone Number: ....
Email Address: ....
Makeup Look: Daytime / Evening / Wedding / Party / Other / (Circle as appropriate).

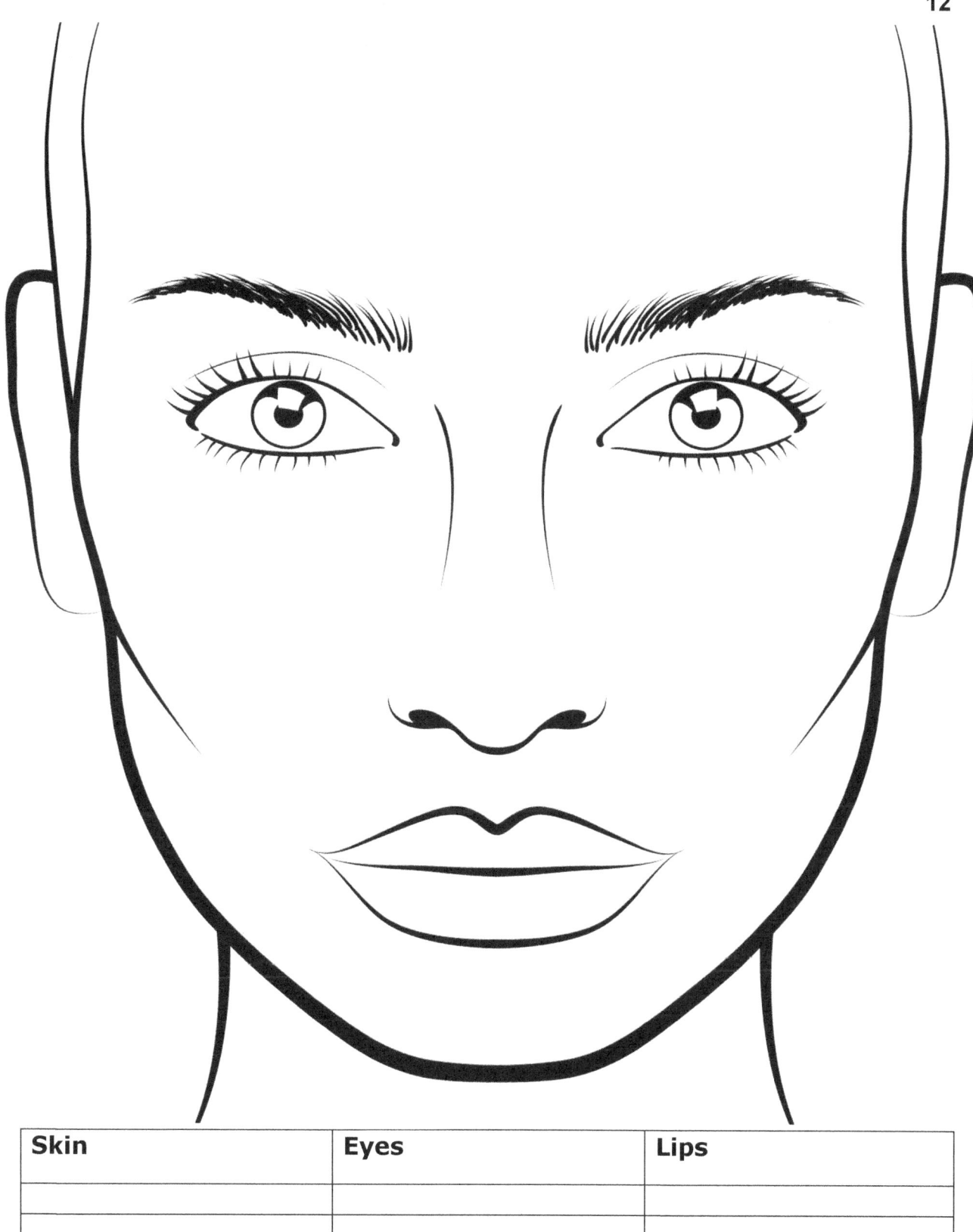

Skin	Eyes	Lips

Client Name: ....
Phone Number: ....
Email Address: ....
Makeup Look: Daytime / Evening / Wedding / Party / Other / (Circle as appropriate).

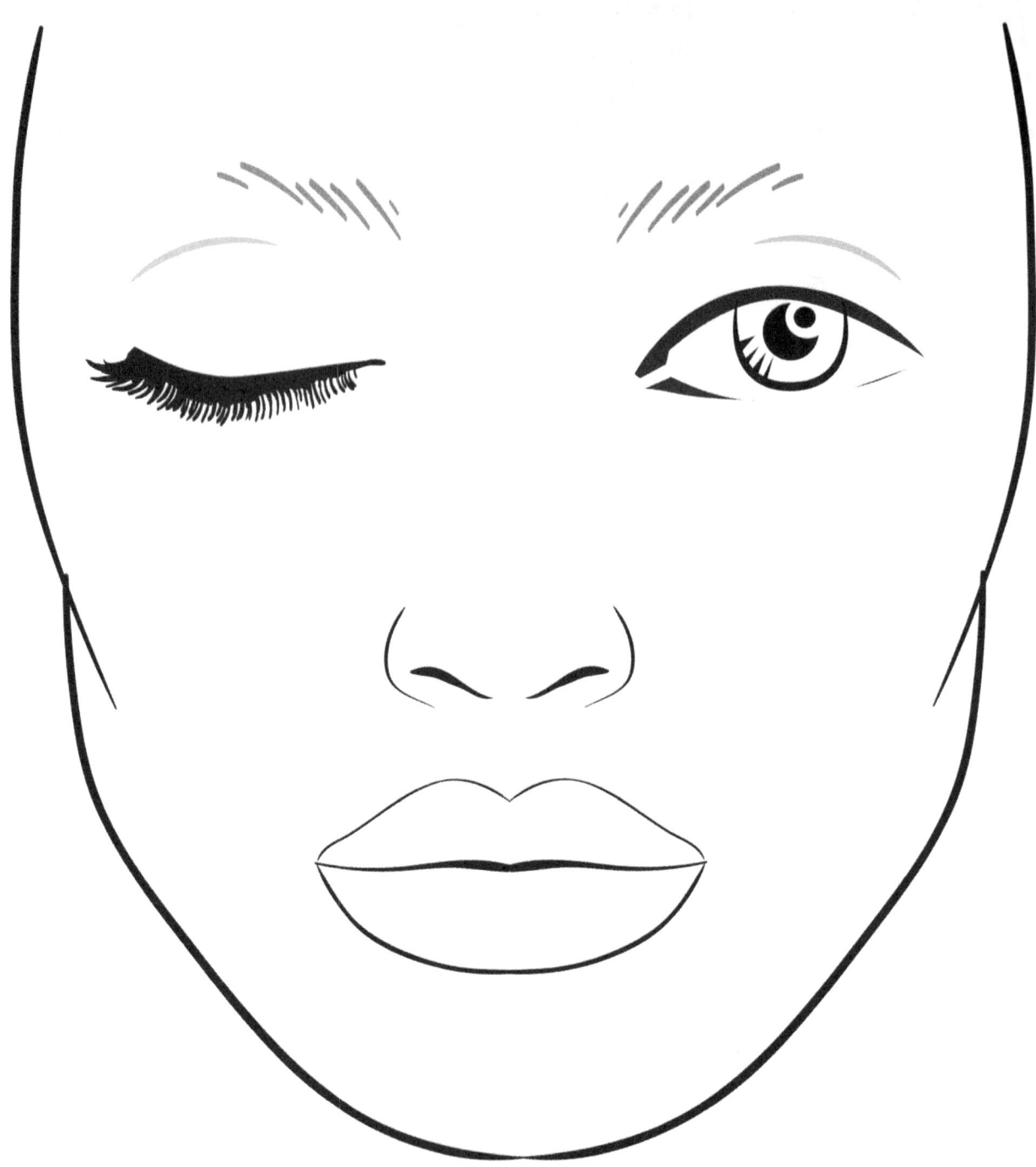

Skin	Eyes	Lips

Client Name: ....
Phone Number: ....
Email Address: ....
Makeup Look: Daytime / Evening / Wedding / Party / Other / (Circle as appropriate).

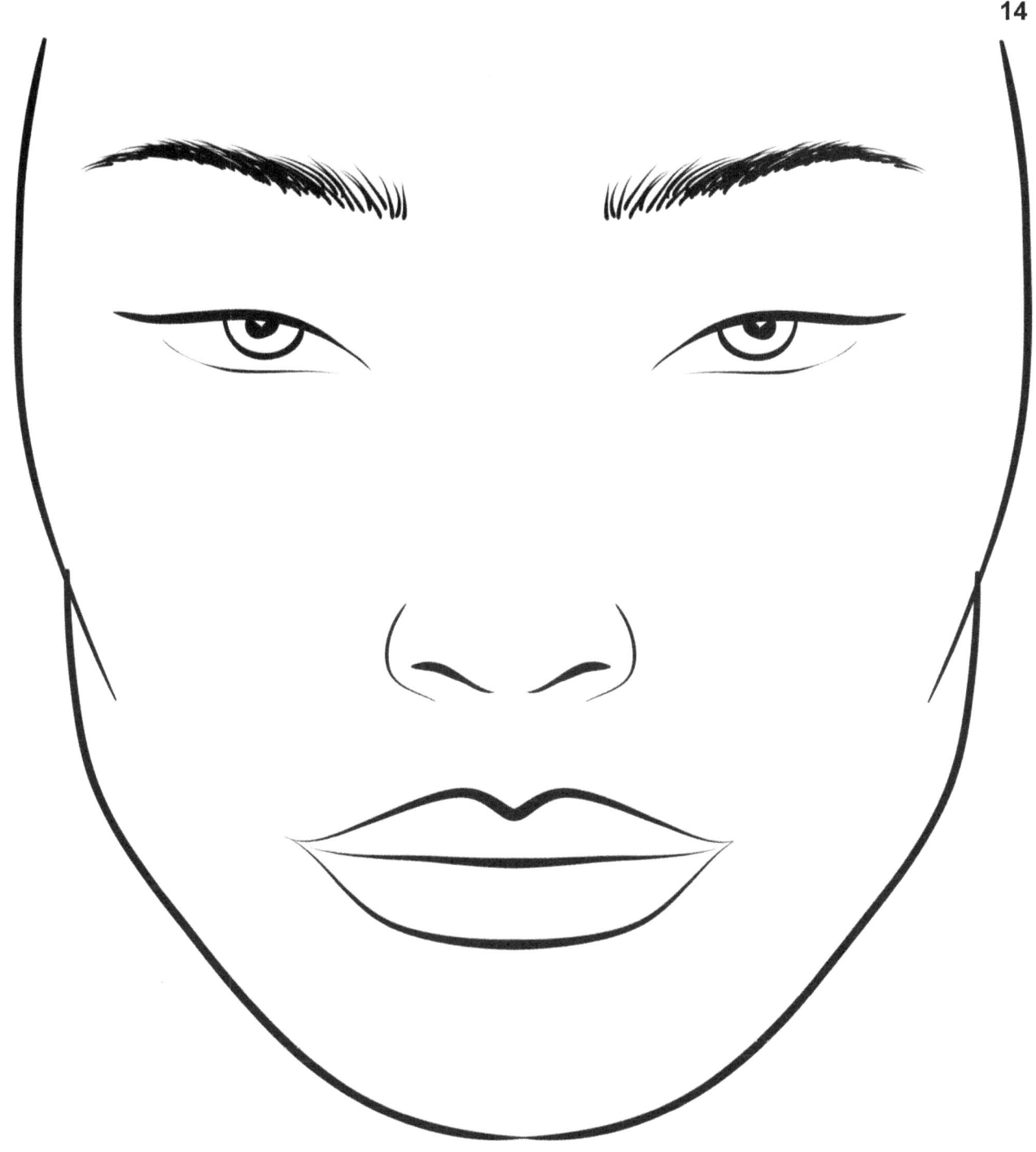

Skin	Eyes	Lips

Client Name: ....

Phone Number: ....

Email Address: ....

Makeup Look: Daytime / Evening / Wedding / Party / Other / (Circle as appropriate).

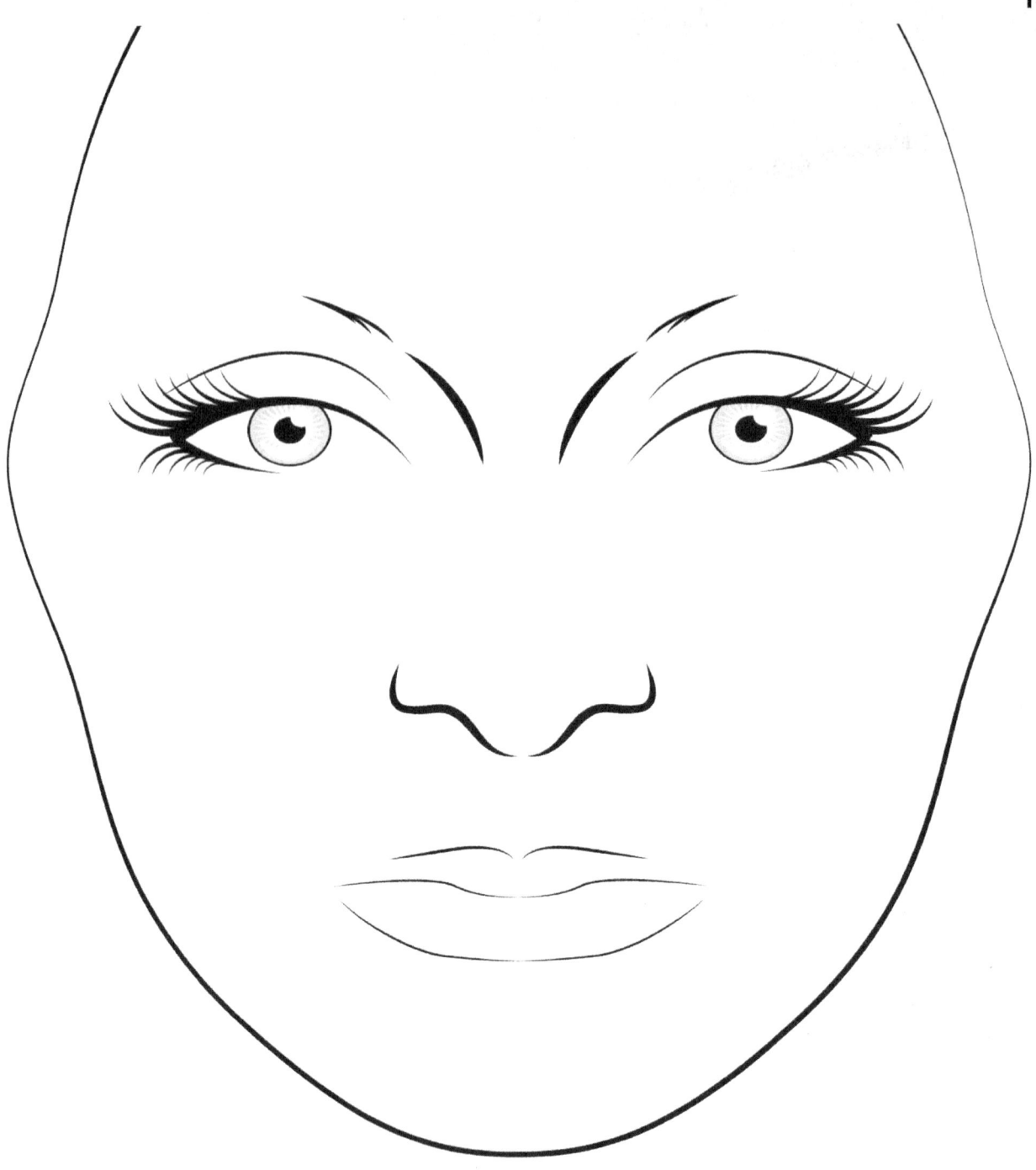

Skin	Eyes	Lips

Client Name: ....
Phone Number: ....
Email Address: ....
Makeup Look: Daytime / Evening / Wedding / Party / Other / (Circle as appropriate).

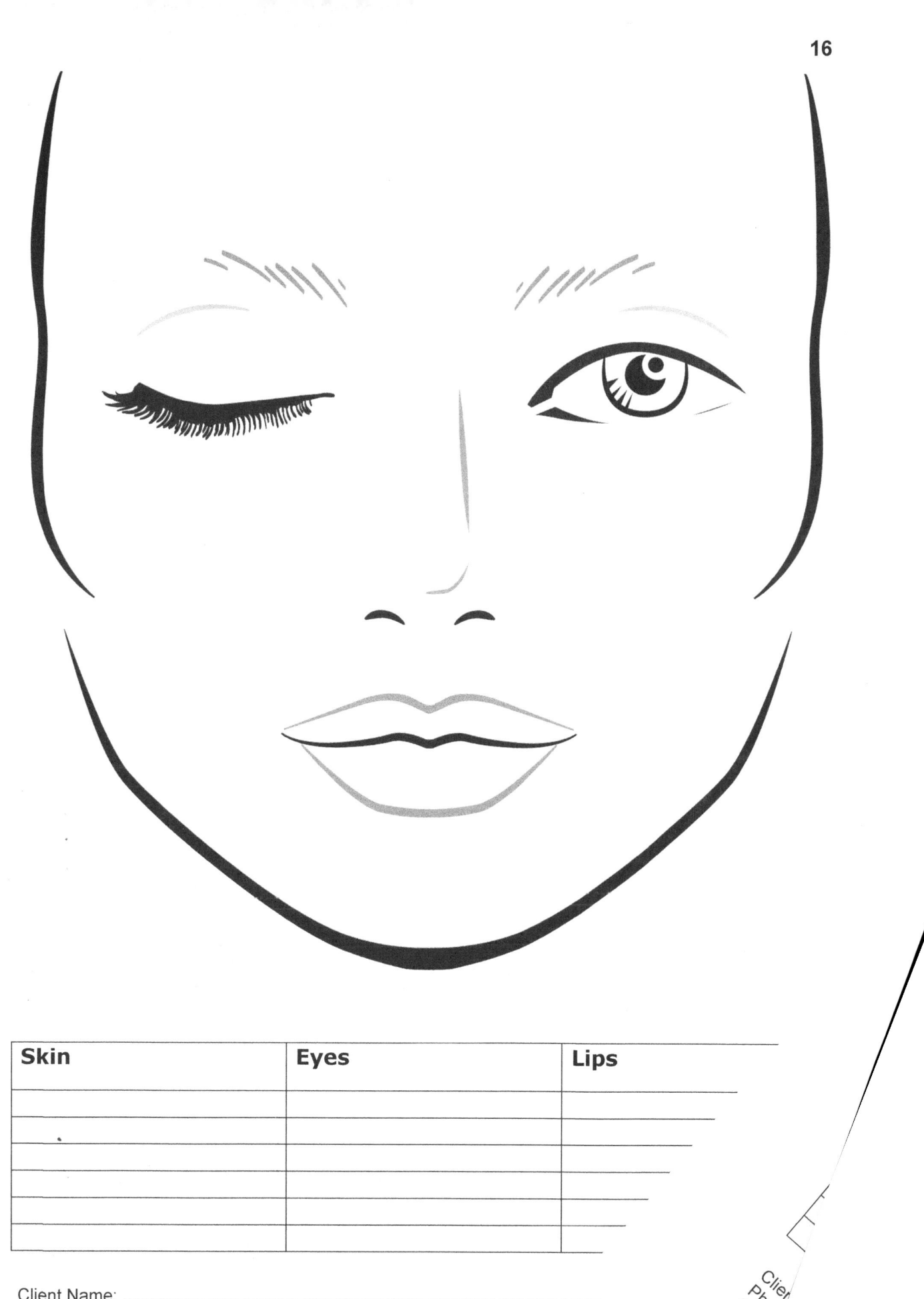

Skin	Eyes	Lips

Client Name: ....
Phone Number: ....
Email Address: ....
Makeup Look: Daytime / Evening / Wedding / Party / Other / (Circle as appropriate).

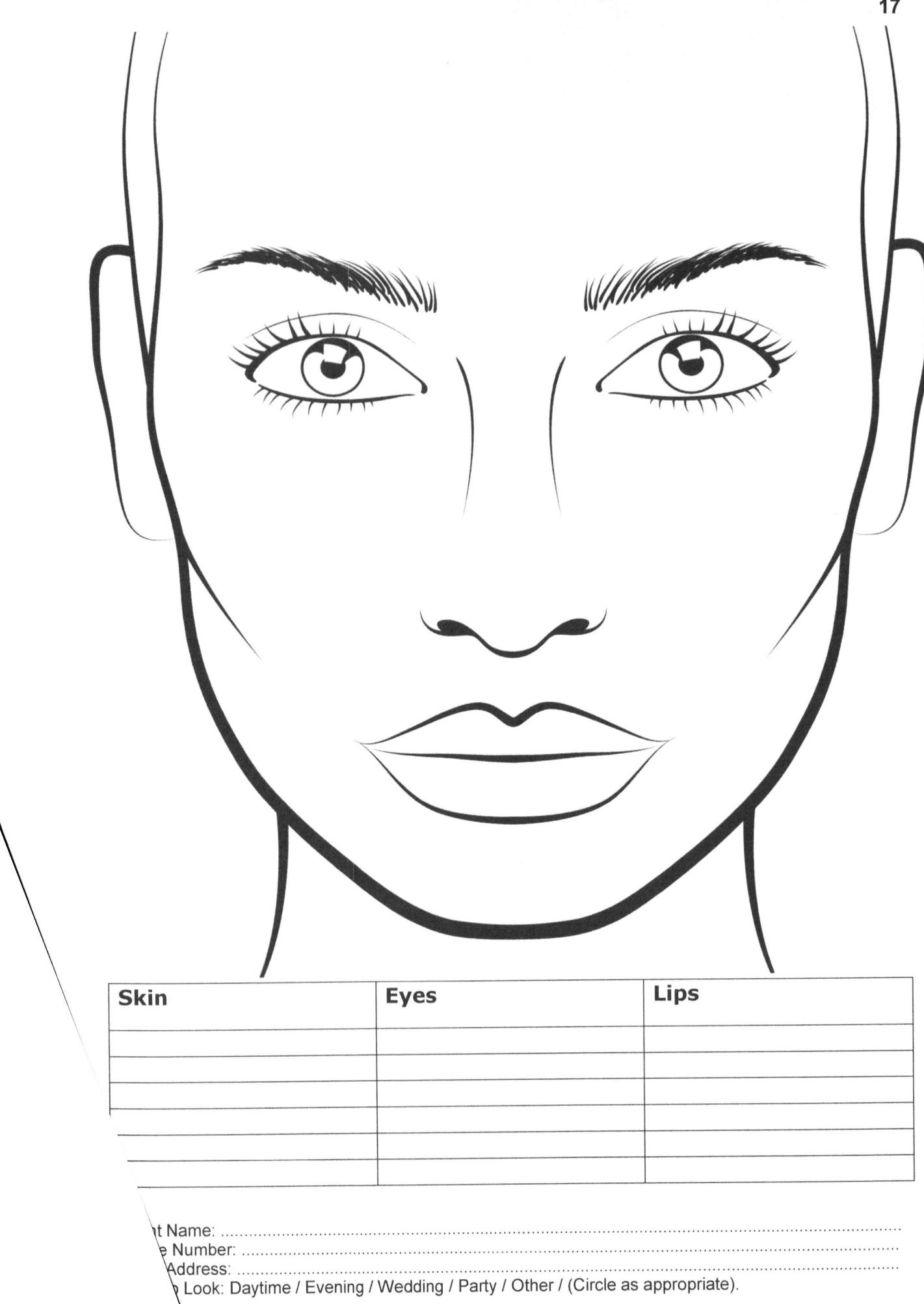

Skin	Eyes	Lips

t Name: ....
e Number: ....
Address: ....
Look: Daytime / Evening / Wedding / Party / Other / (Circle as appropriate).

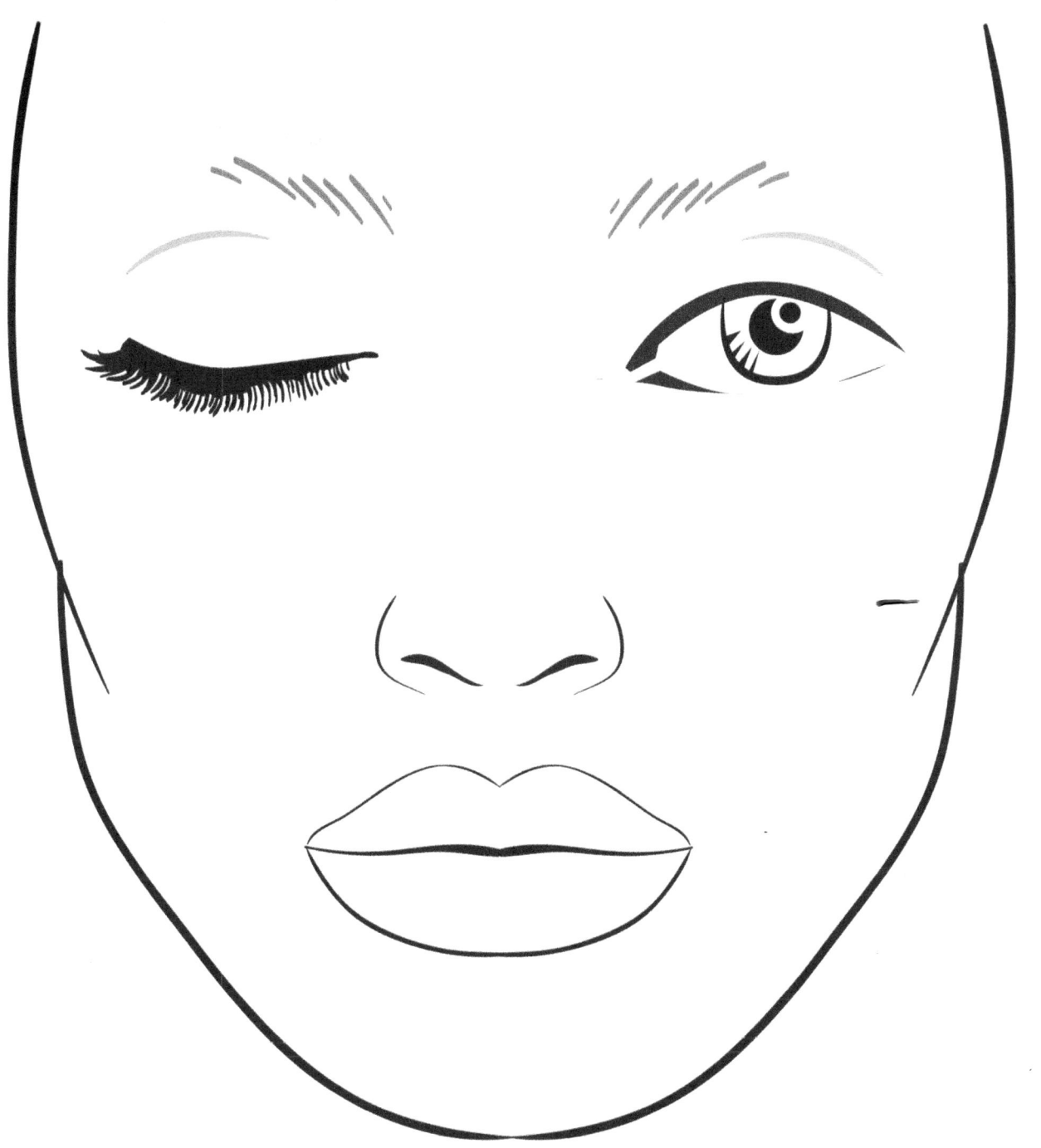

Skin	Eyes	Lips

Client Name: ....
Phone Number: ....
Email Address: ....
Makeup Look: Daytime / Evening / Wedding / Party / Other / (Circle as appropriate).

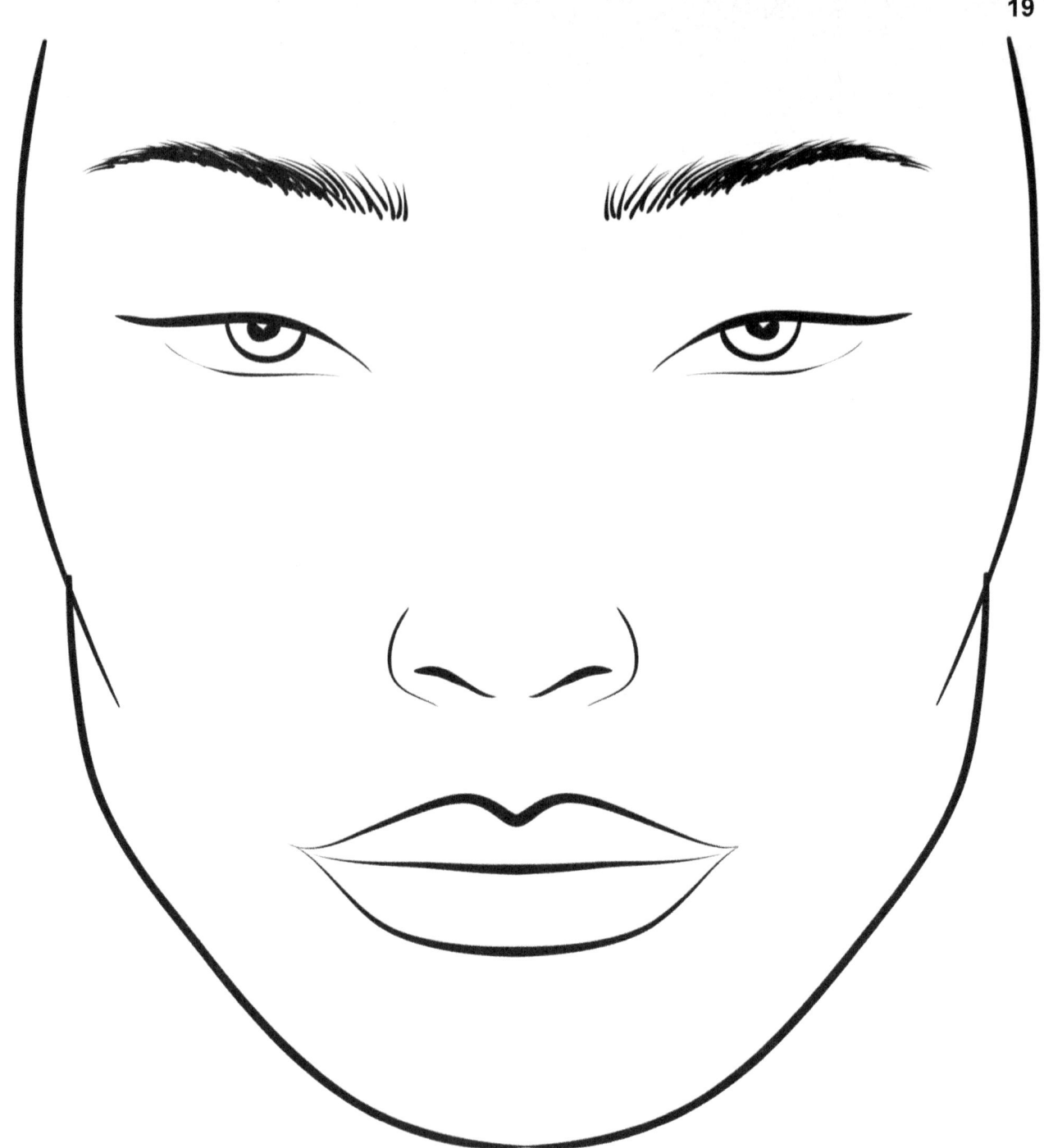

Skin	Eyes	Lips

Client Name: ....
Phone Number: ....
Email Address: ....
Makeup Look: Daytime / Evening / Wedding / Party / Other / (Circle as appropriate).

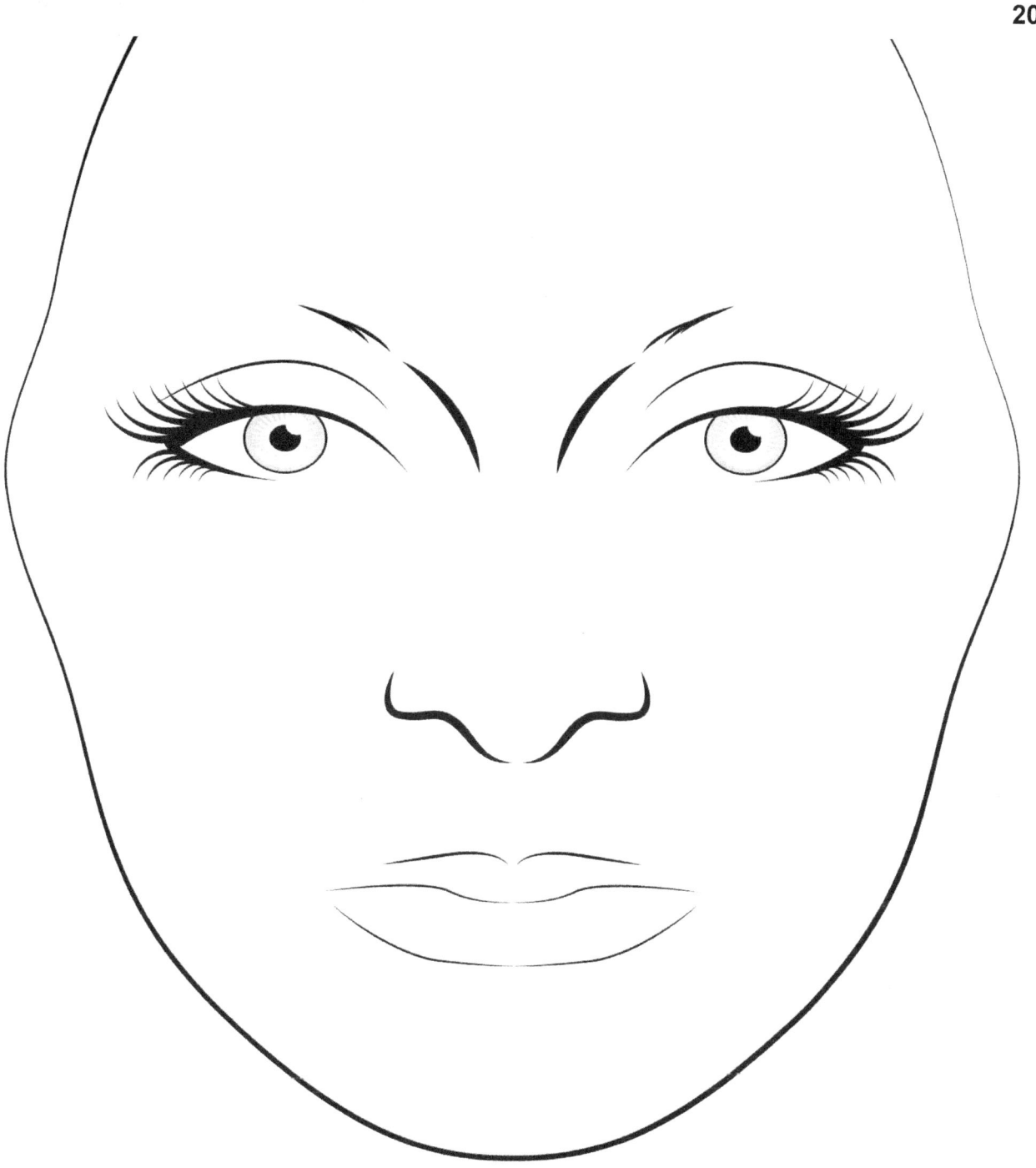

Skin	Eyes	Lips

Client Name: ....
Phone Number: ....
Email Address: ....
Makeup Look: Daytime / Evening / Wedding / Party / Other / (Circle as appropriate).

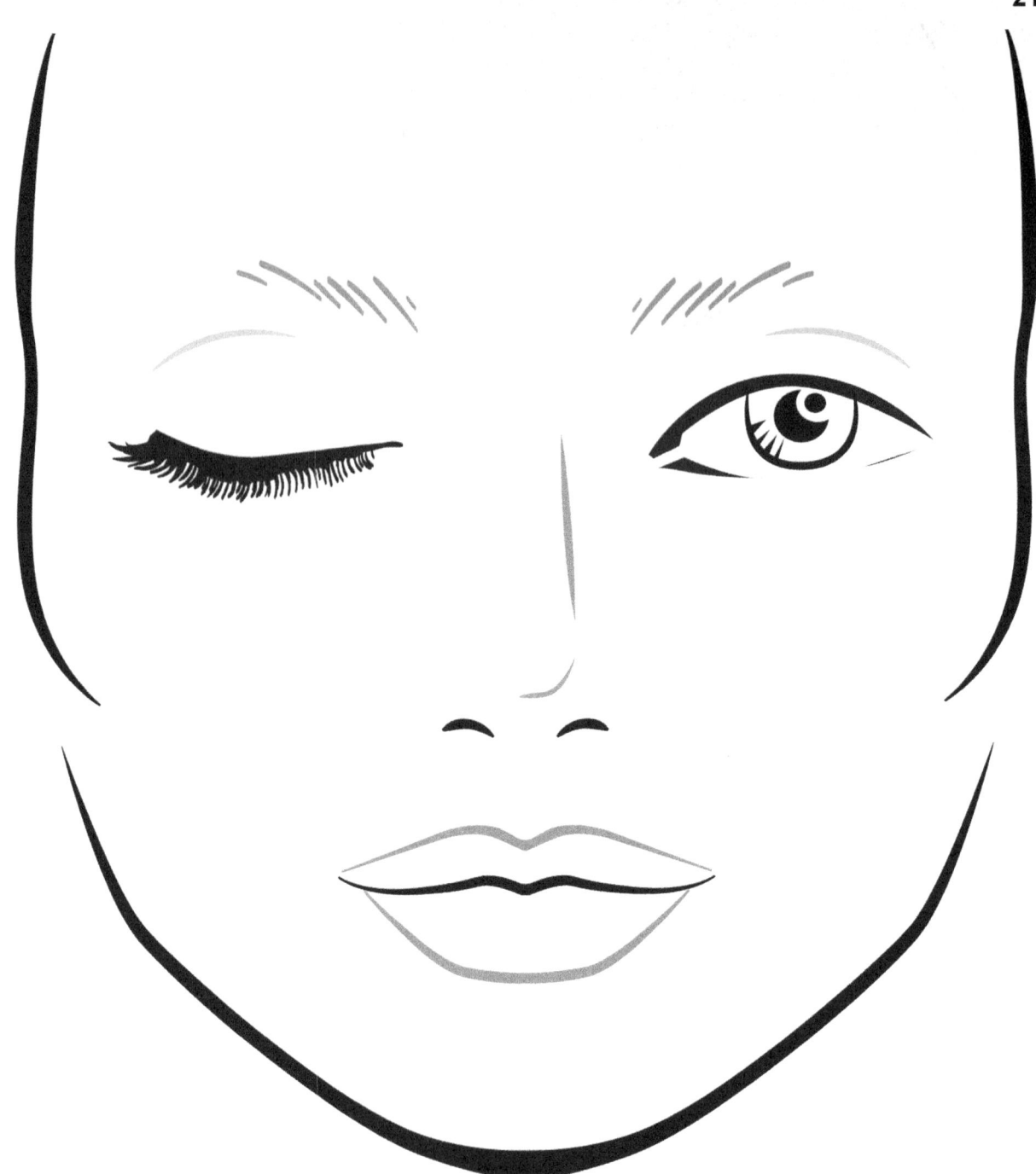

Skin	Eyes	Lips

Client Name: ....
Phone Number: ....
Email Address: ....
Makeup Look: Daytime / Evening / Wedding / Party / Other / (Circle as appropriate).

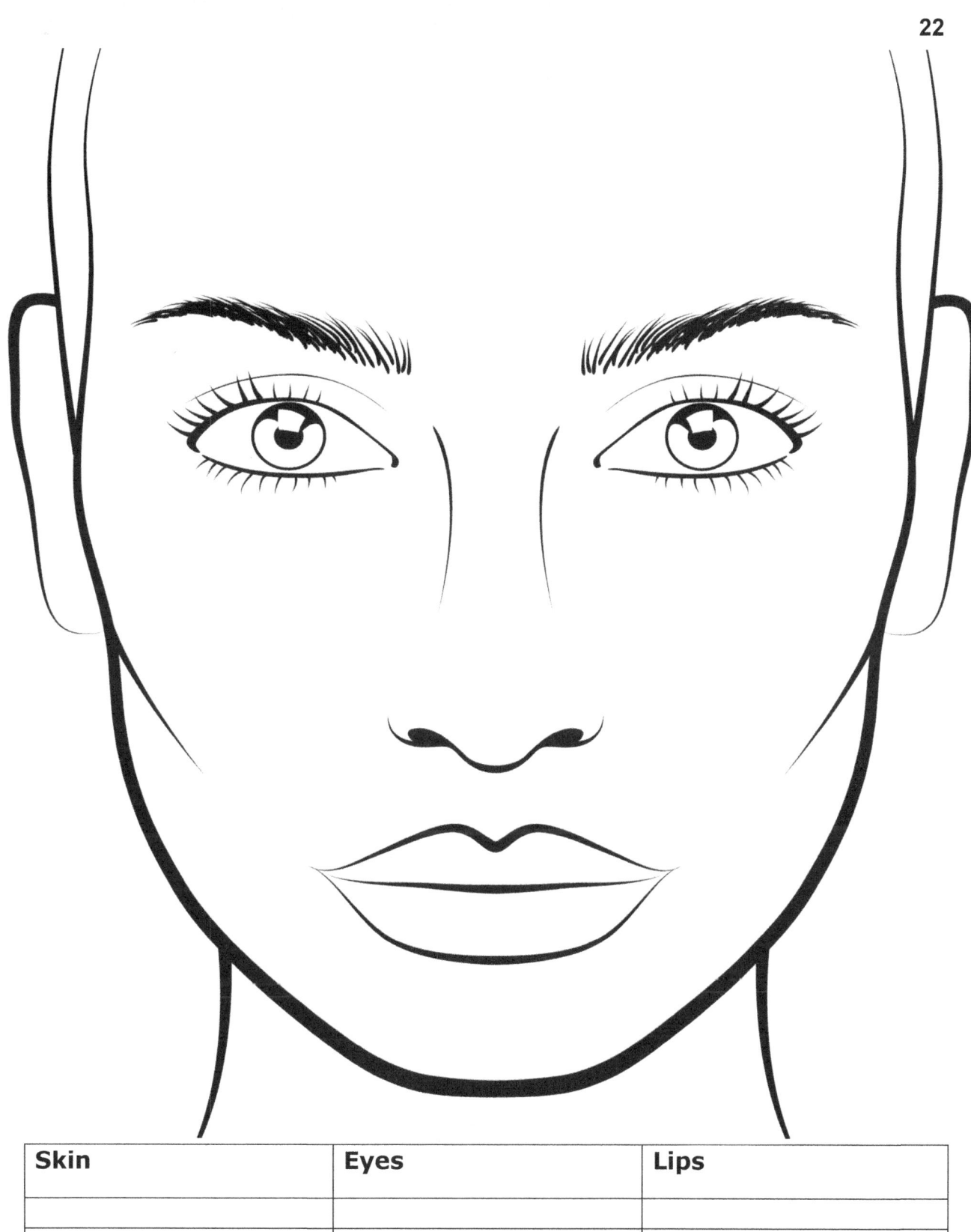

Skin	Eyes	Lips

Client Name: ....
Phone Number: ....
Email Address: ....
Makeup Look: Daytime / Evening / Wedding / Party / Other / (Circle as appropriate).

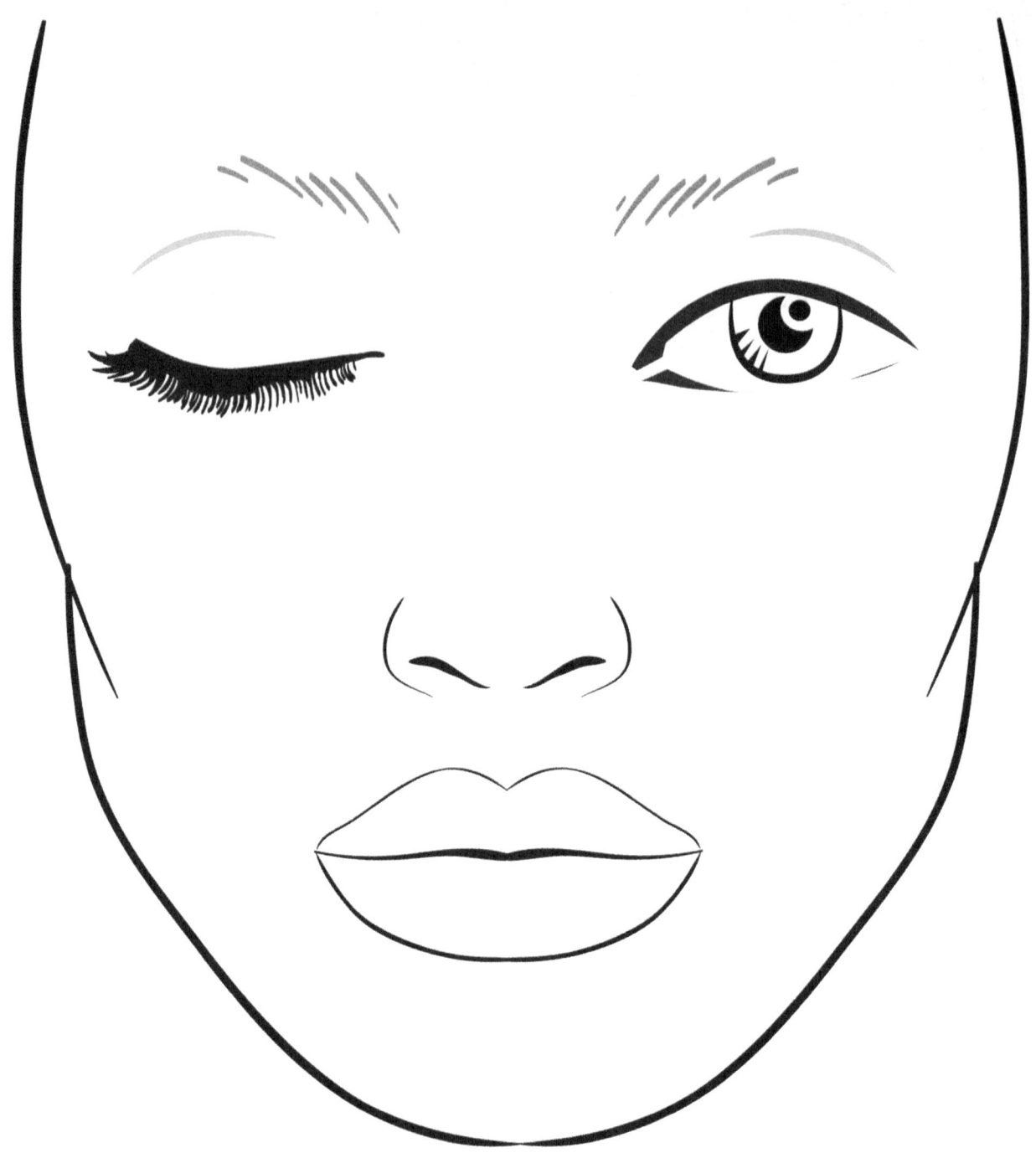

Skin	Eyes	Lips

Client Name: ....
Phone Number: ....
Email Address: ....
Makeup Look: Daytime / Evening / Wedding / Party / Other / (Circle as appropriate).

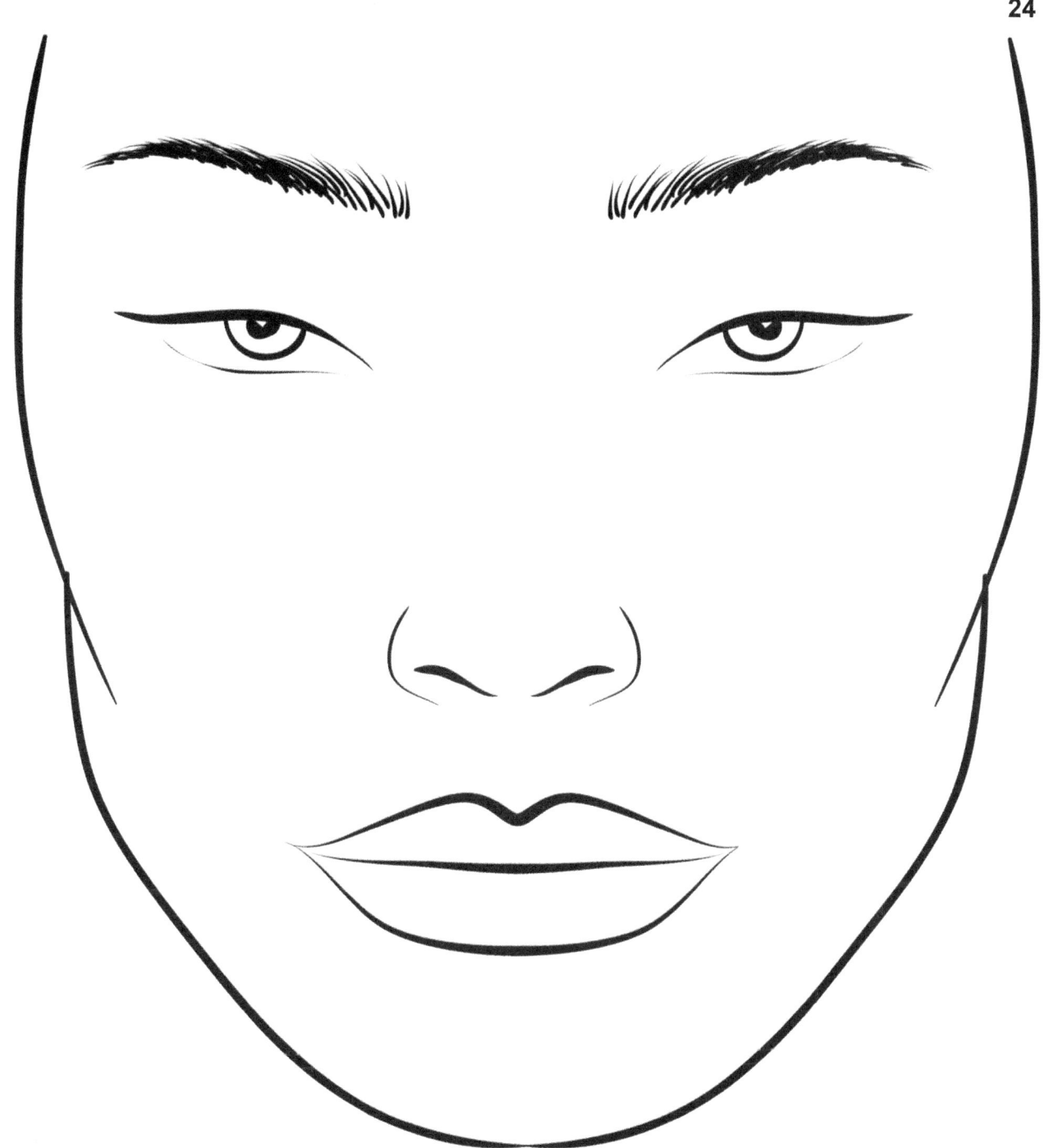

Skin	Eyes	Lips

Client Name: ....
Phone Number: ....
Email Address: ....
Makeup Look: Daytime / Evening / Wedding / Party / Other / (Circle as appropriate).

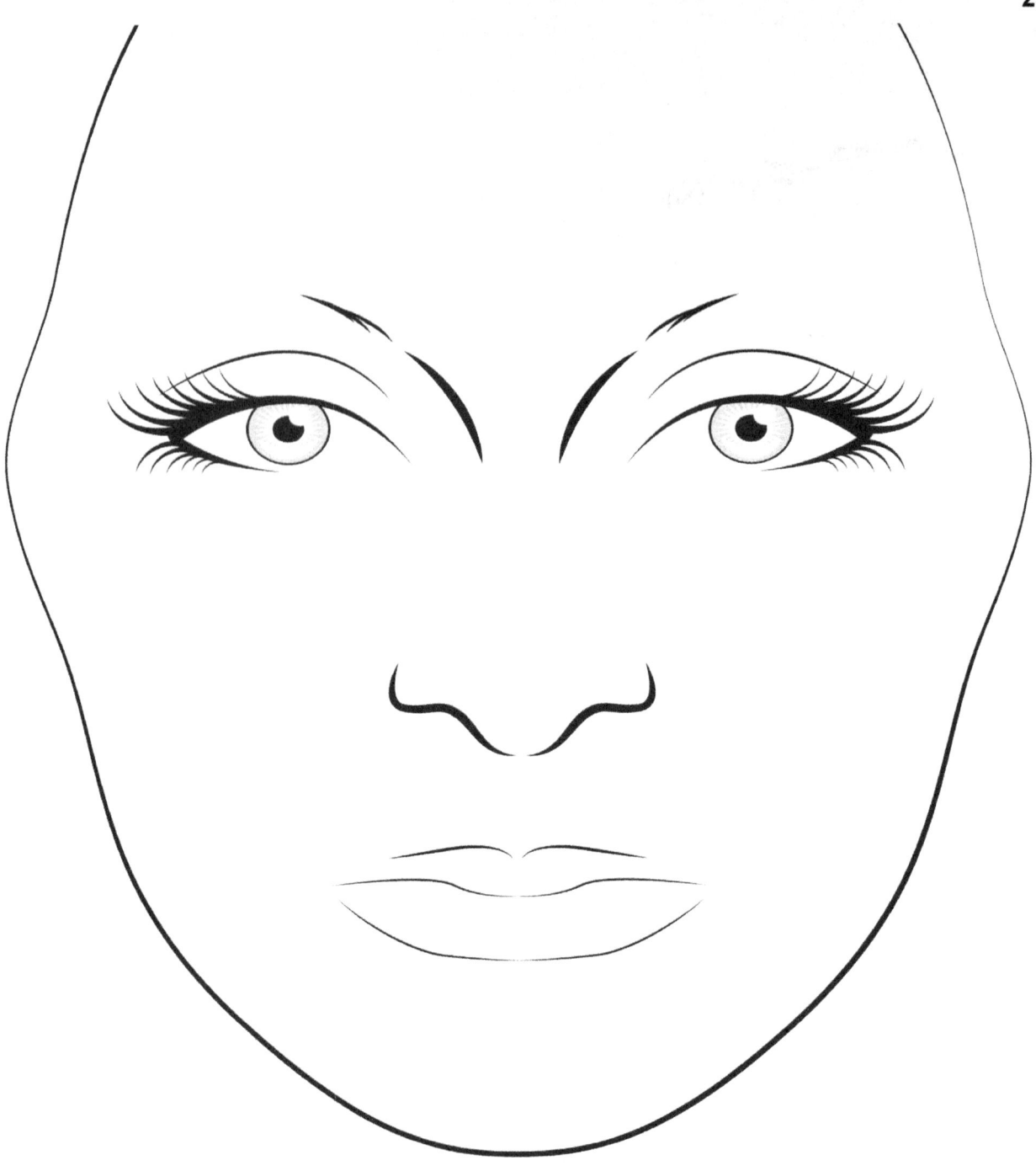

Skin	Eyes	Lips

Client Name: ....
Phone Number: ....
Email Address: ....
Makeup Look: Daytime / Evening / Wedding / Party / Other / (Circle as appropriate).

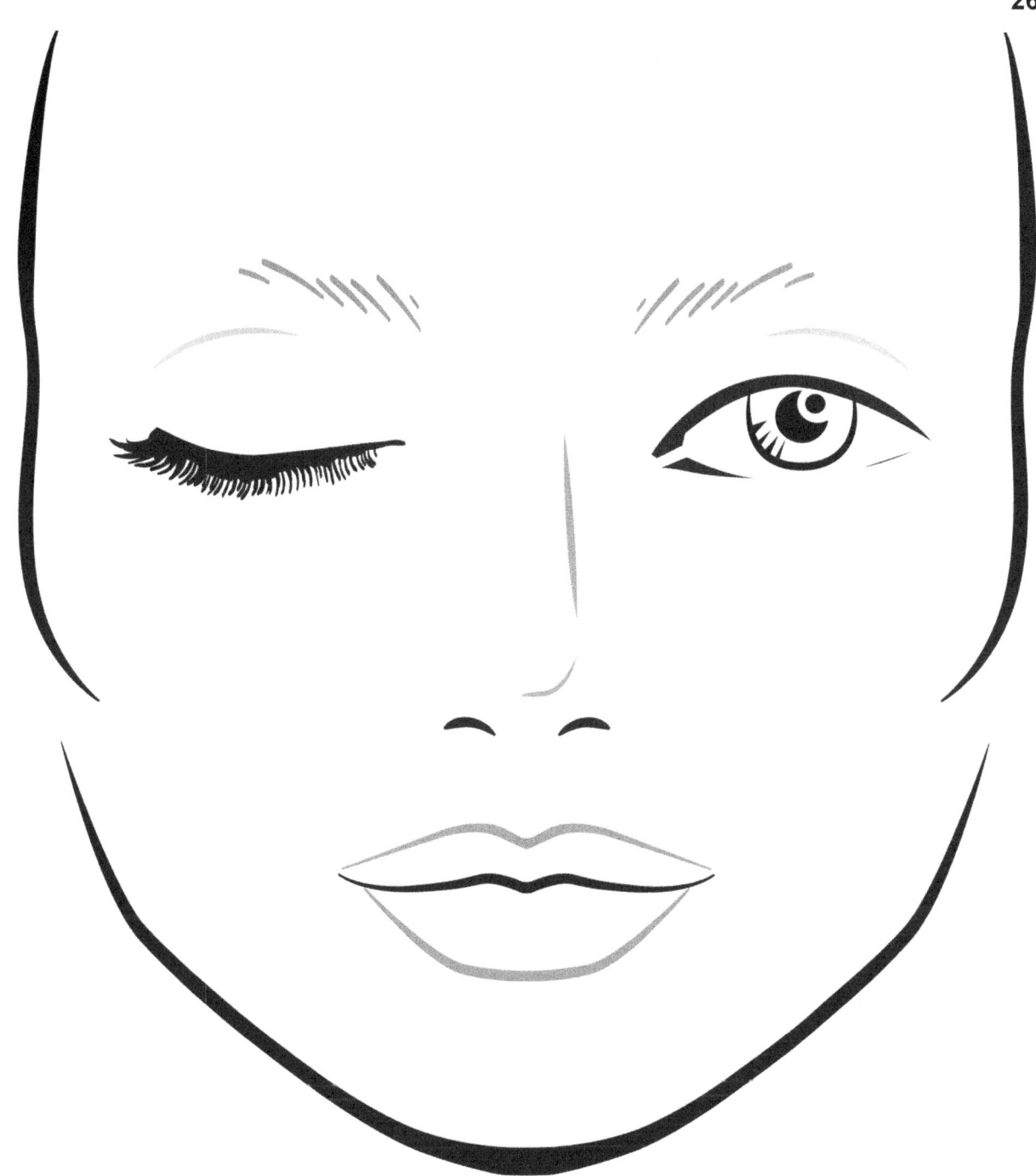

Skin	Eyes	Lips

Client Name: ....
Phone Number: ....
Email Address: ....
Makeup Look: Daytime / Evening / Wedding / Party / Other / (Circle as appropriate).

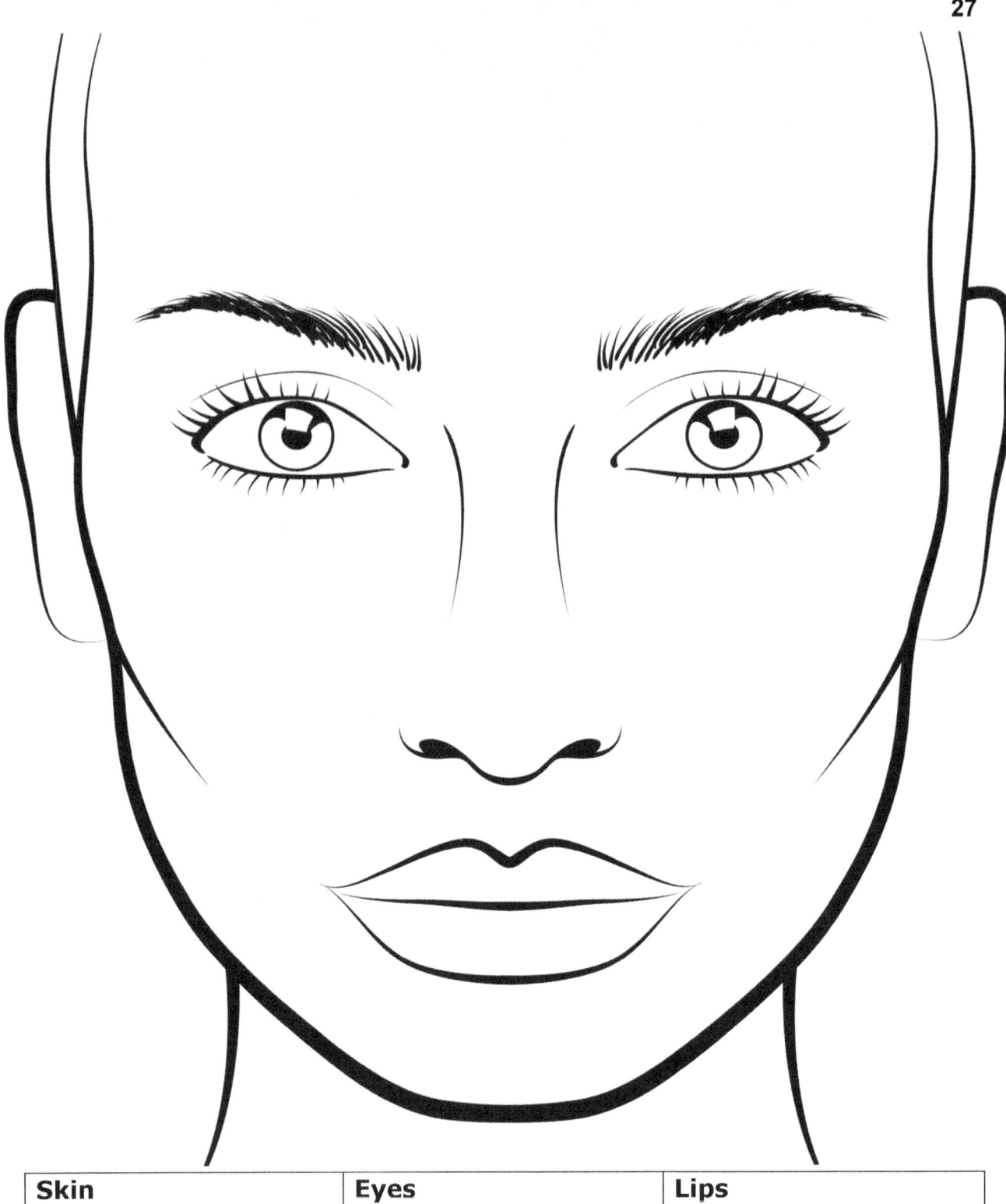

Skin	Eyes	Lips

Client Name: ....
Phone Number: ....
Email Address: ....
Makeup Look: Daytime / Evening / Wedding / Party / Other / (Circle as appropriate).

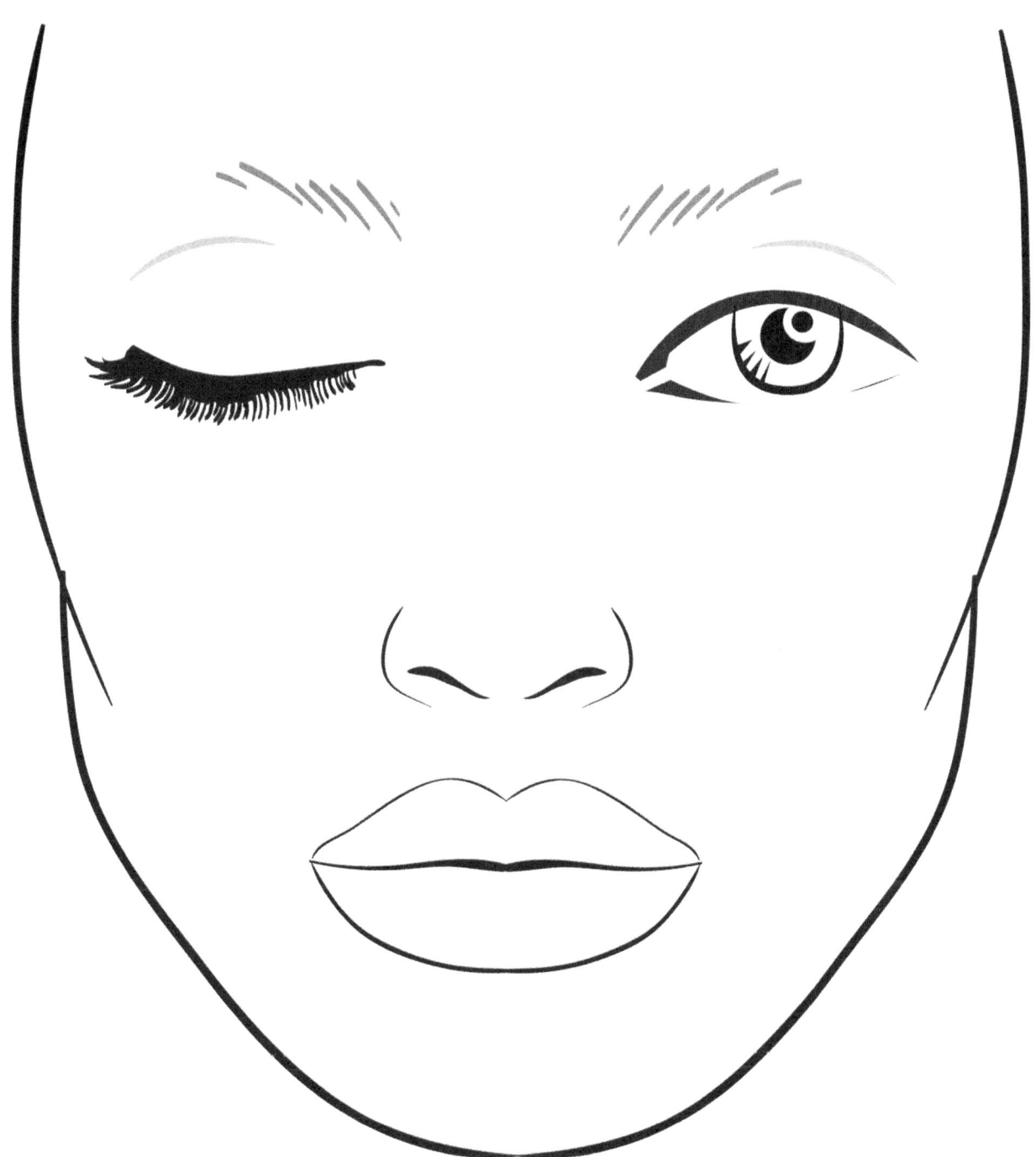

Skin	Eyes	Lips

Client Name: ....

Phone Number: ....

Email Address: ....

Makeup Look: Daytime / Evening / Wedding / Party / Other / (Circle as appropriate).

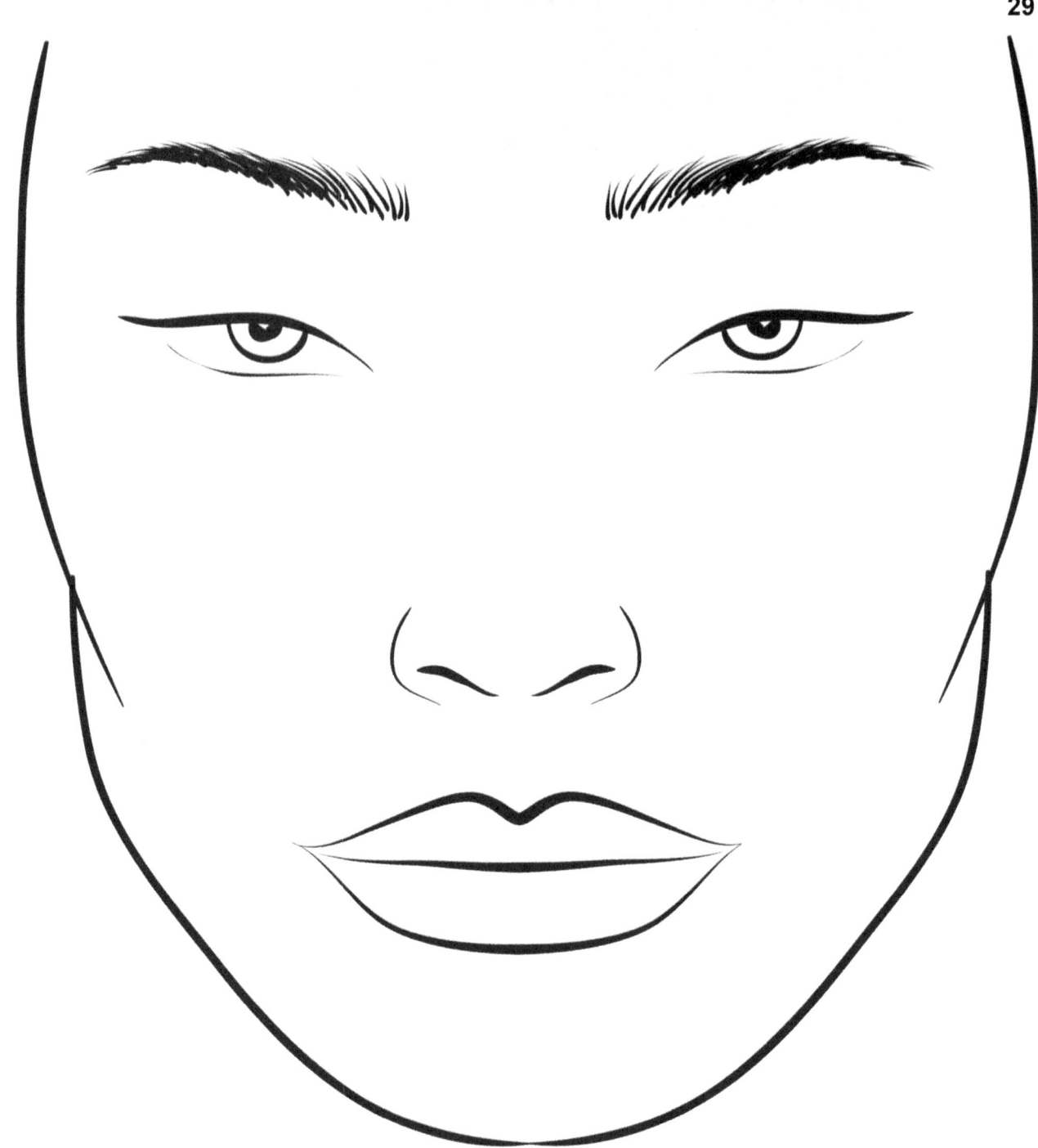

Skin	Eyes	Lips

Client Name: ....
Phone Number: ....
Email Address: ....
Makeup Look: Daytime / Evening / Wedding / Party / Other / (Circle as appropriate).

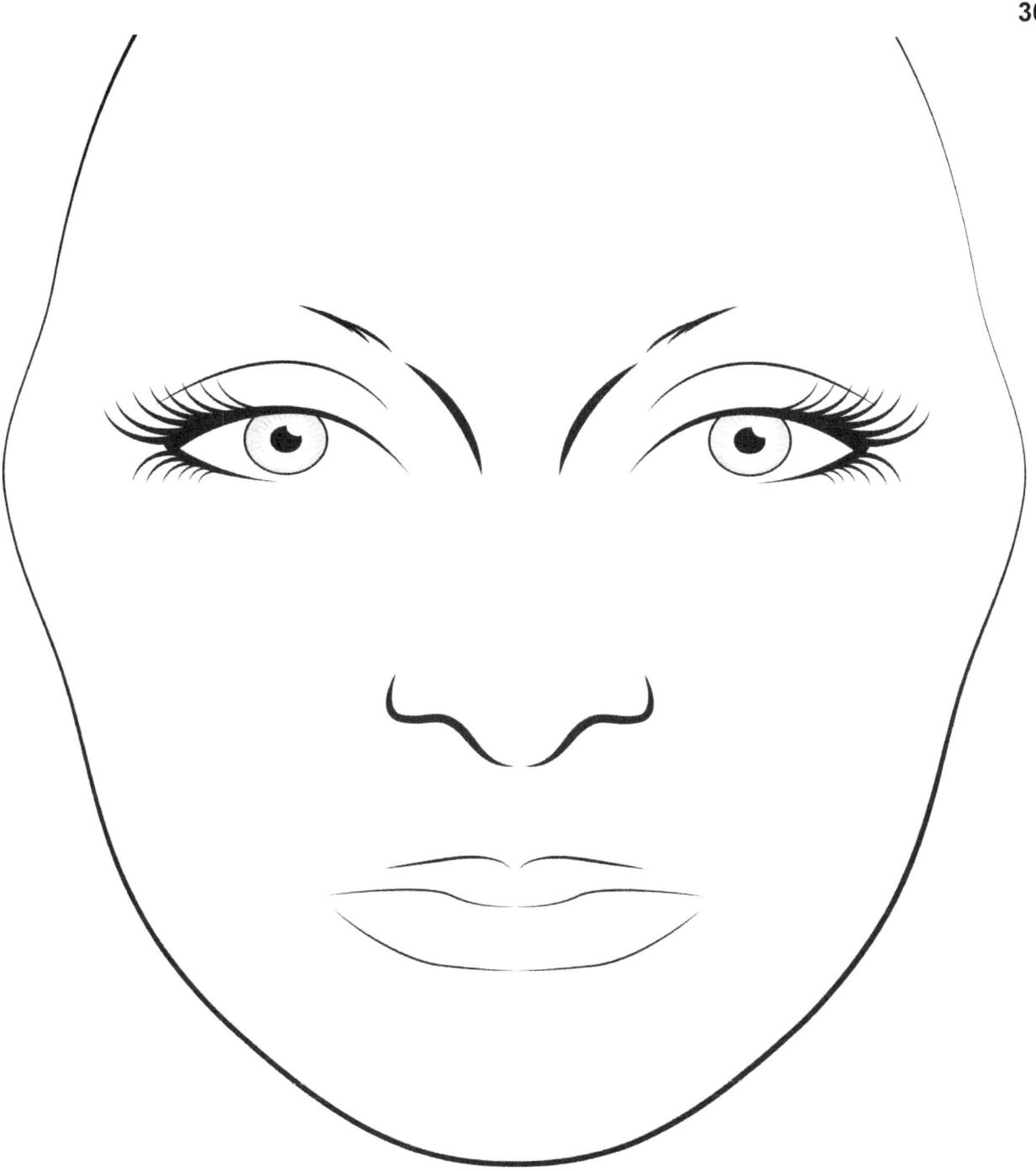

Skin	Eyes	Lips

Client Name: ....
Phone Number: ....
Email Address: ....
Makeup Look: Daytime / Evening / Wedding / Party / Other / (Circle as appropriate).

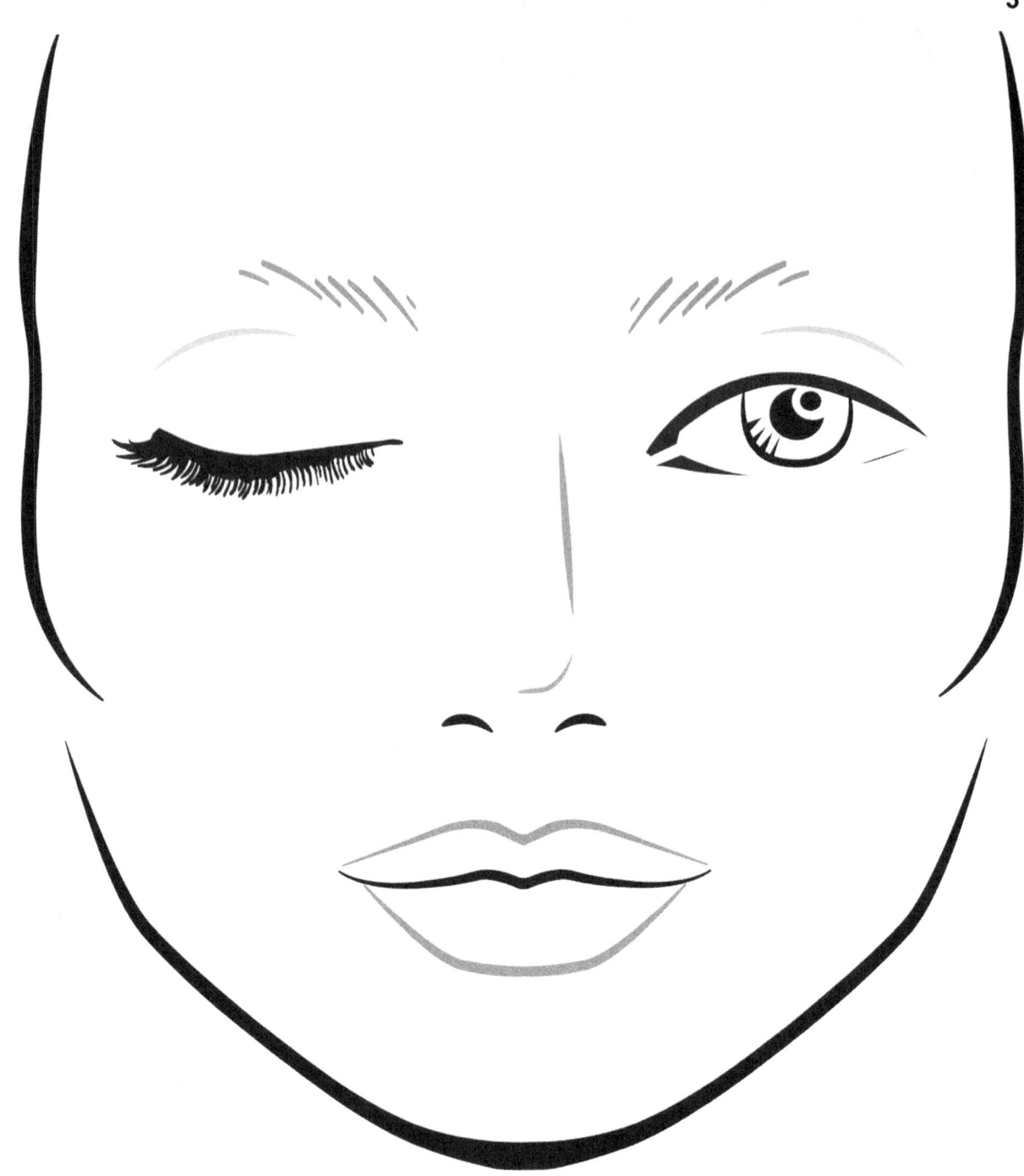

Skin	Eyes	Lips

Client Name: ....
Phone Number: ....
Email Address: ....
Makeup Look: Daytime / Evening / Wedding / Party / Other / (Circle as appropriate).

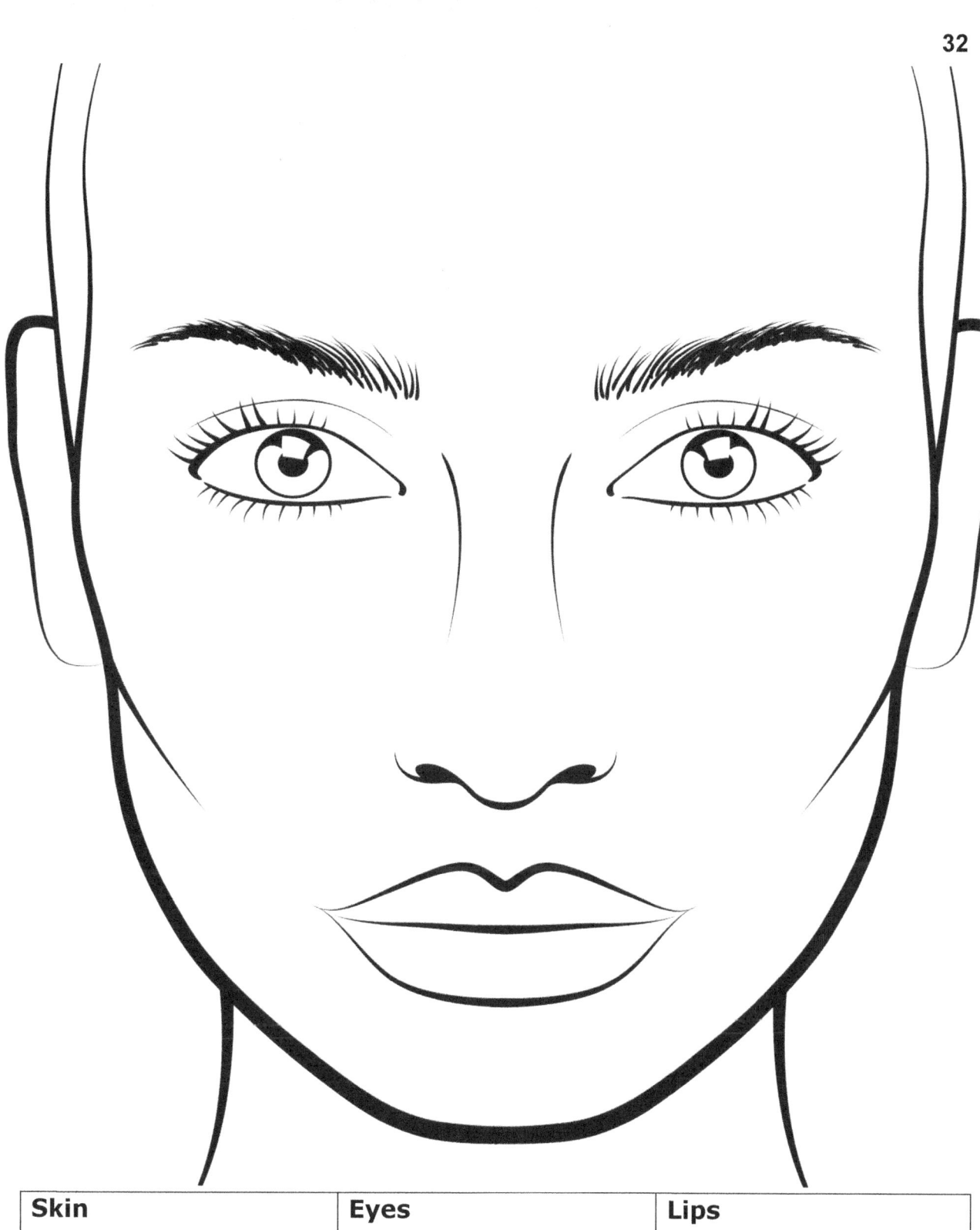

Skin	Eyes	Lips

Client Name: ....
Phone Number: ....
Email Address: ....
Makeup Look: Daytime / Evening / Wedding / Party / Other / (Circle as appropriate).

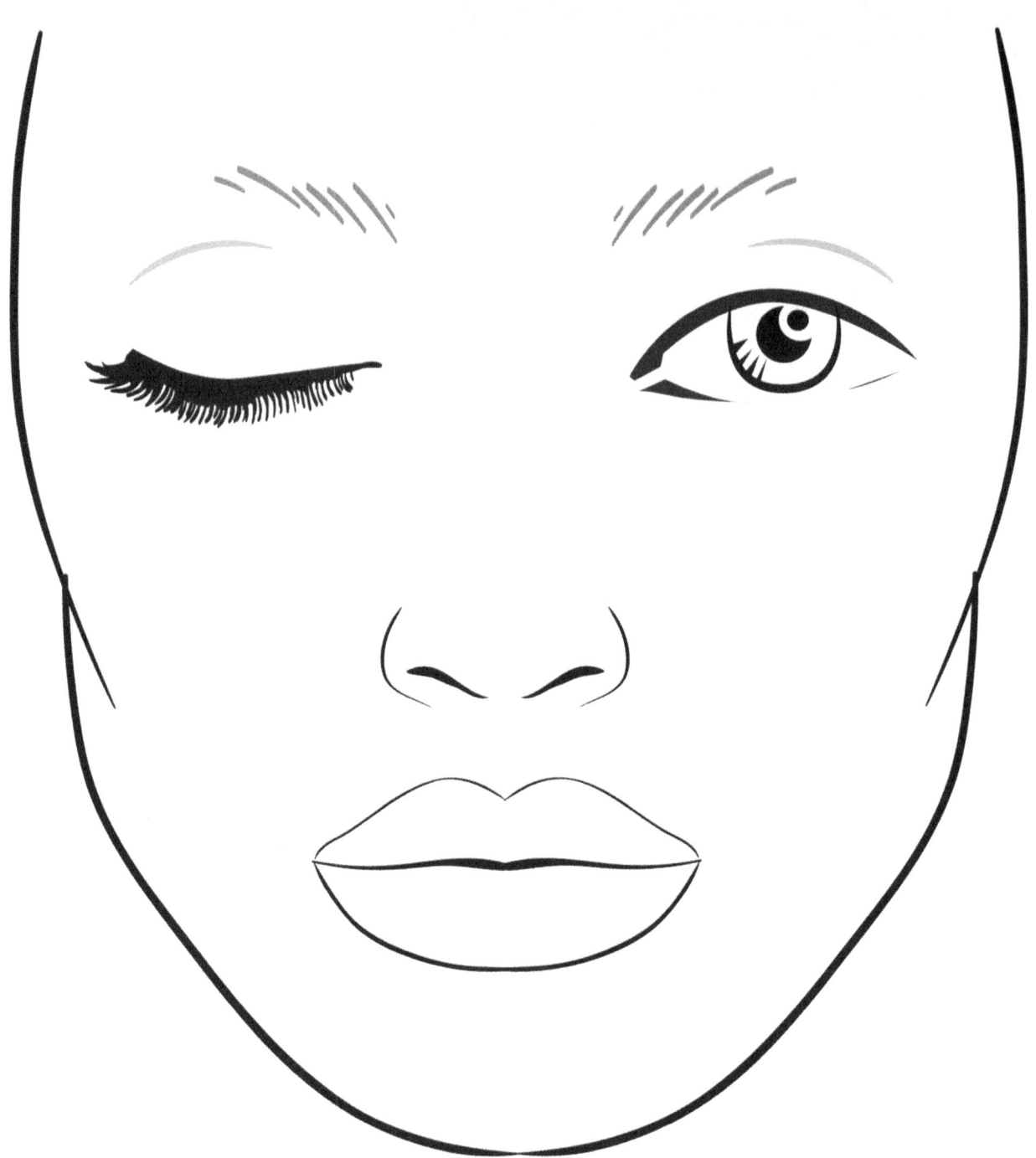

Skin	Eyes	Lips

Client Name: ....
Phone Number: ....
Email Address: ....
Makeup Look: Daytime / Evening / Wedding / Party / Other / (Circle as appropriate).

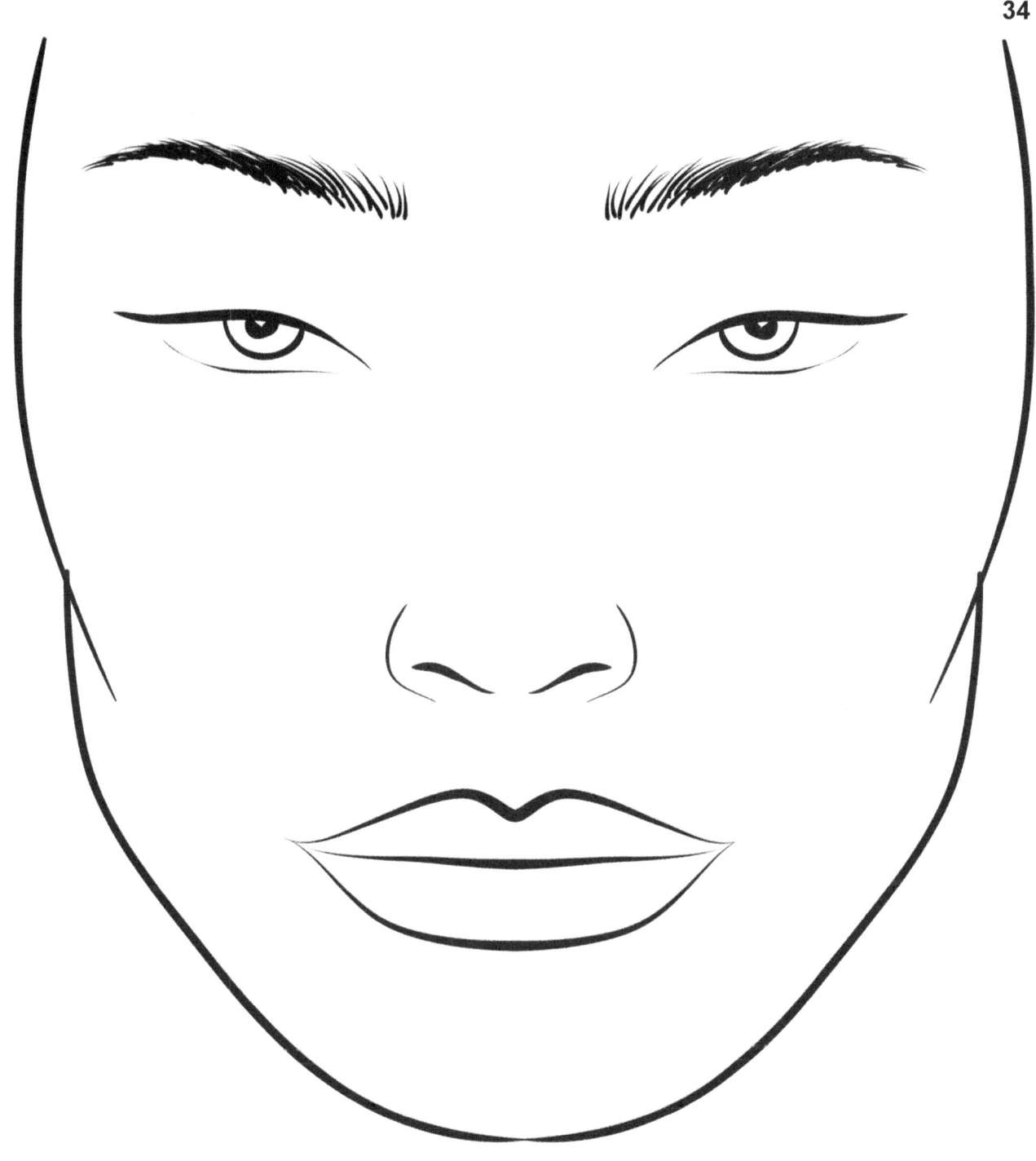

Skin	Eyes	Lips

Client Name: ....
Phone Number: ....
Email Address: ....
Makeup Look: Daytime / Evening / Wedding / Party / Other / (Circle as appropriate).

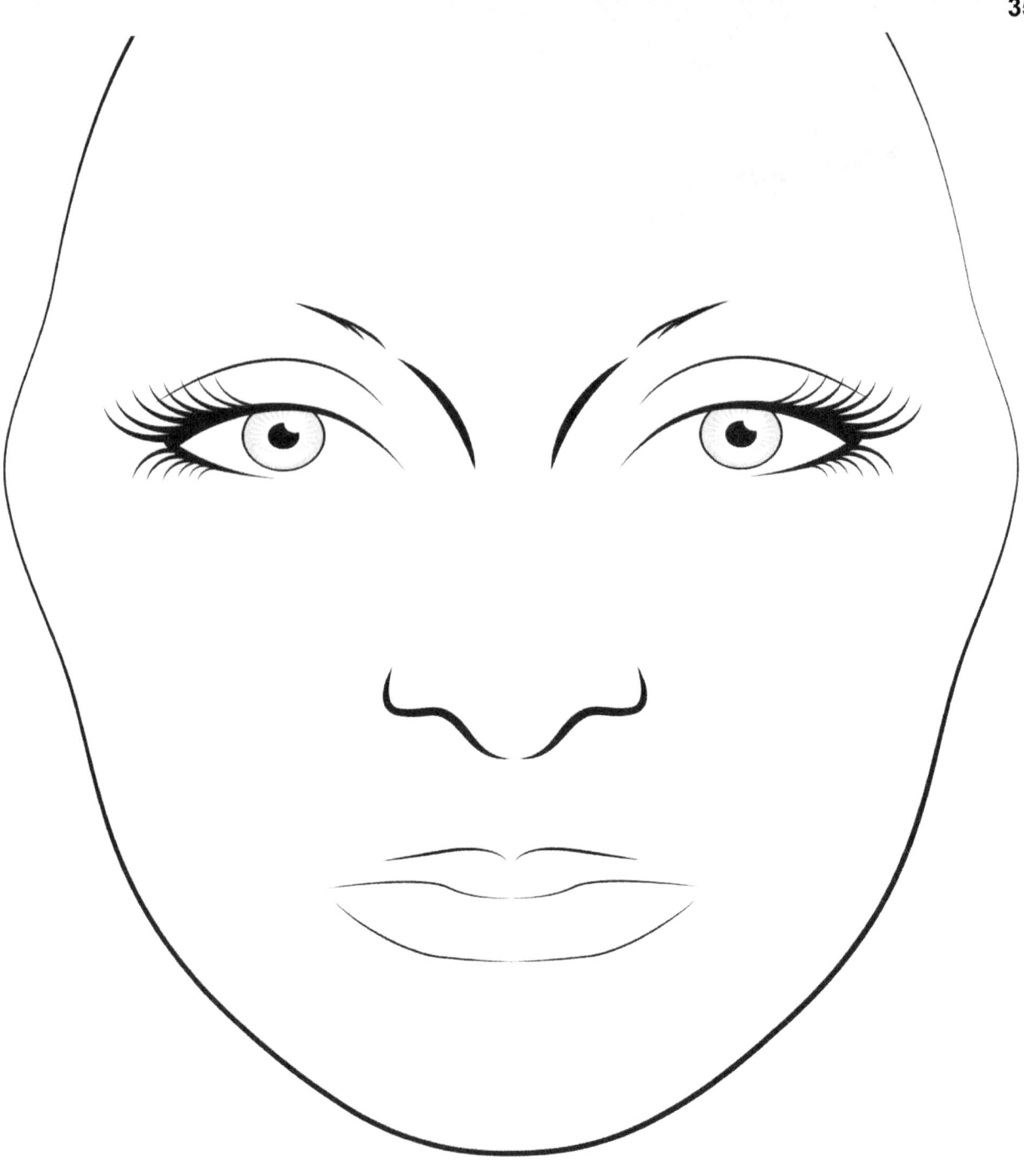

Skin	Eyes	Lips

Client Name: ....

Phone Number: ....

Email Address: ....

Makeup Look: Daytime / Evening / Wedding / Party / Other / (Circle as appropriate).

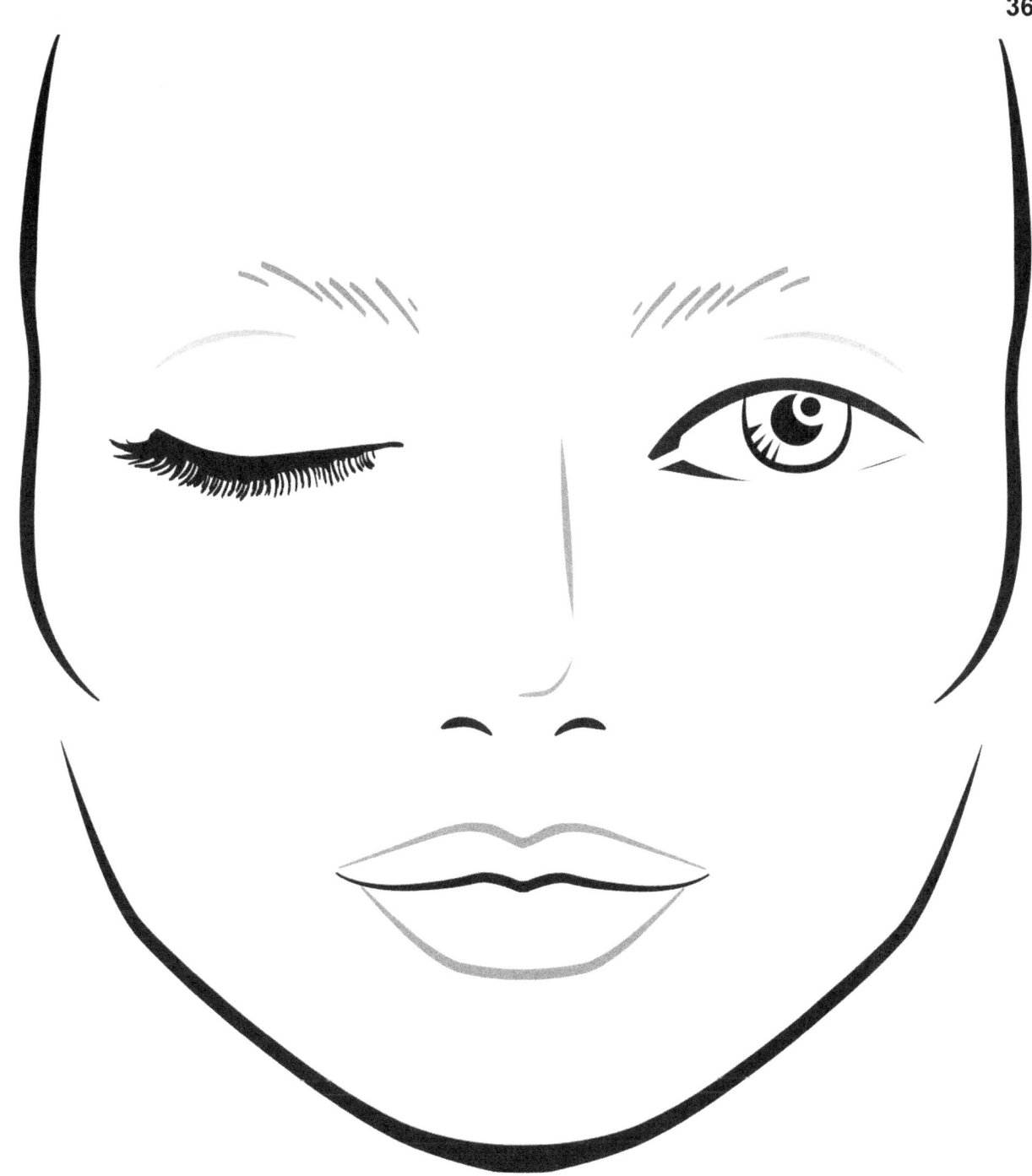

Skin	Eyes	Lips

Client Name: ....
Phone Number: ....
Email Address: ....
Makeup Look: Daytime / Evening / Wedding / Party / Other / (Circle as appropriate).

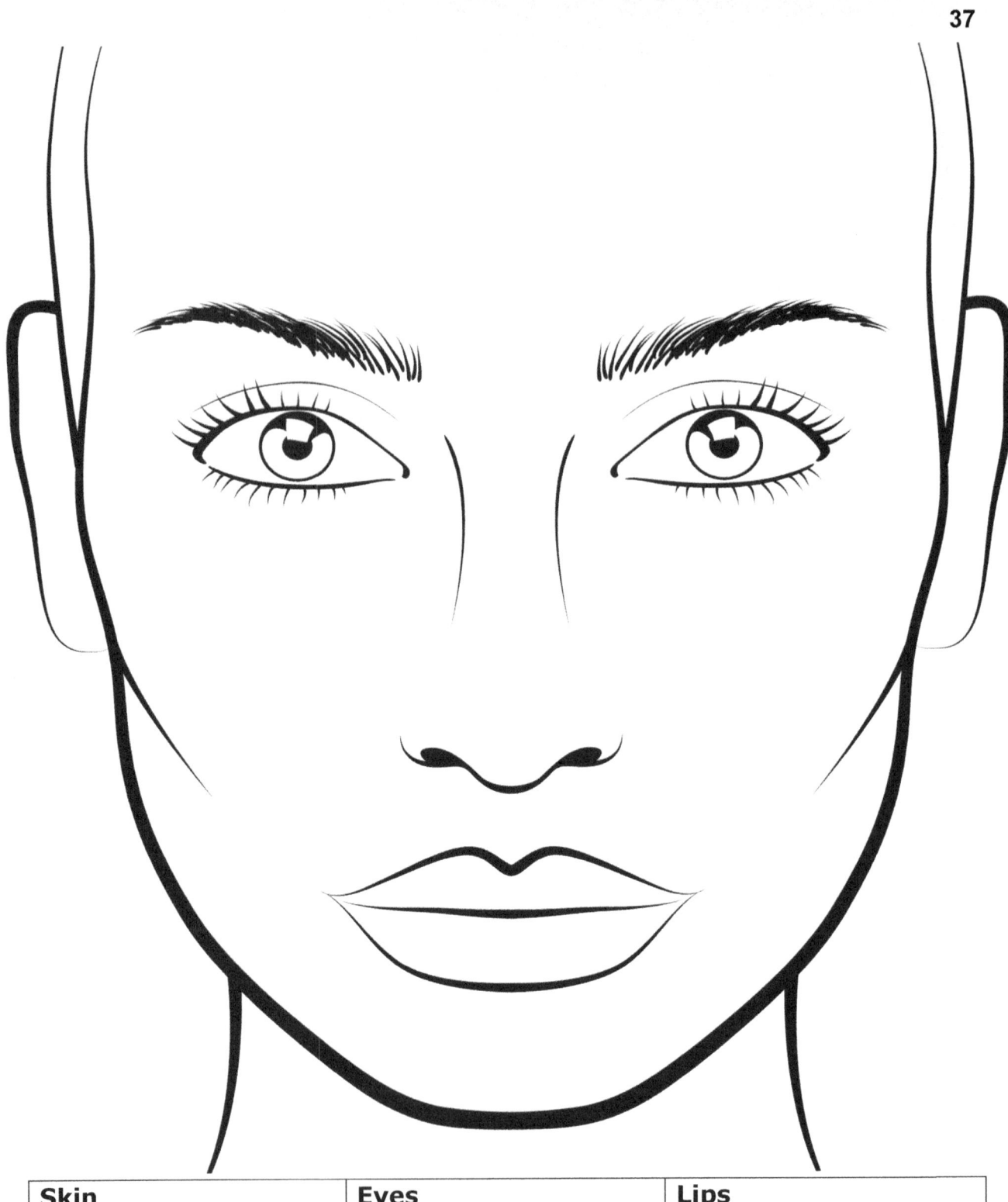

Skin	Eyes	Lips

Client Name: ....
Phone Number: ....
Email Address: ....
Makeup Look: Daytime / Evening / Wedding / Party / Other / (Circle as appropriate).

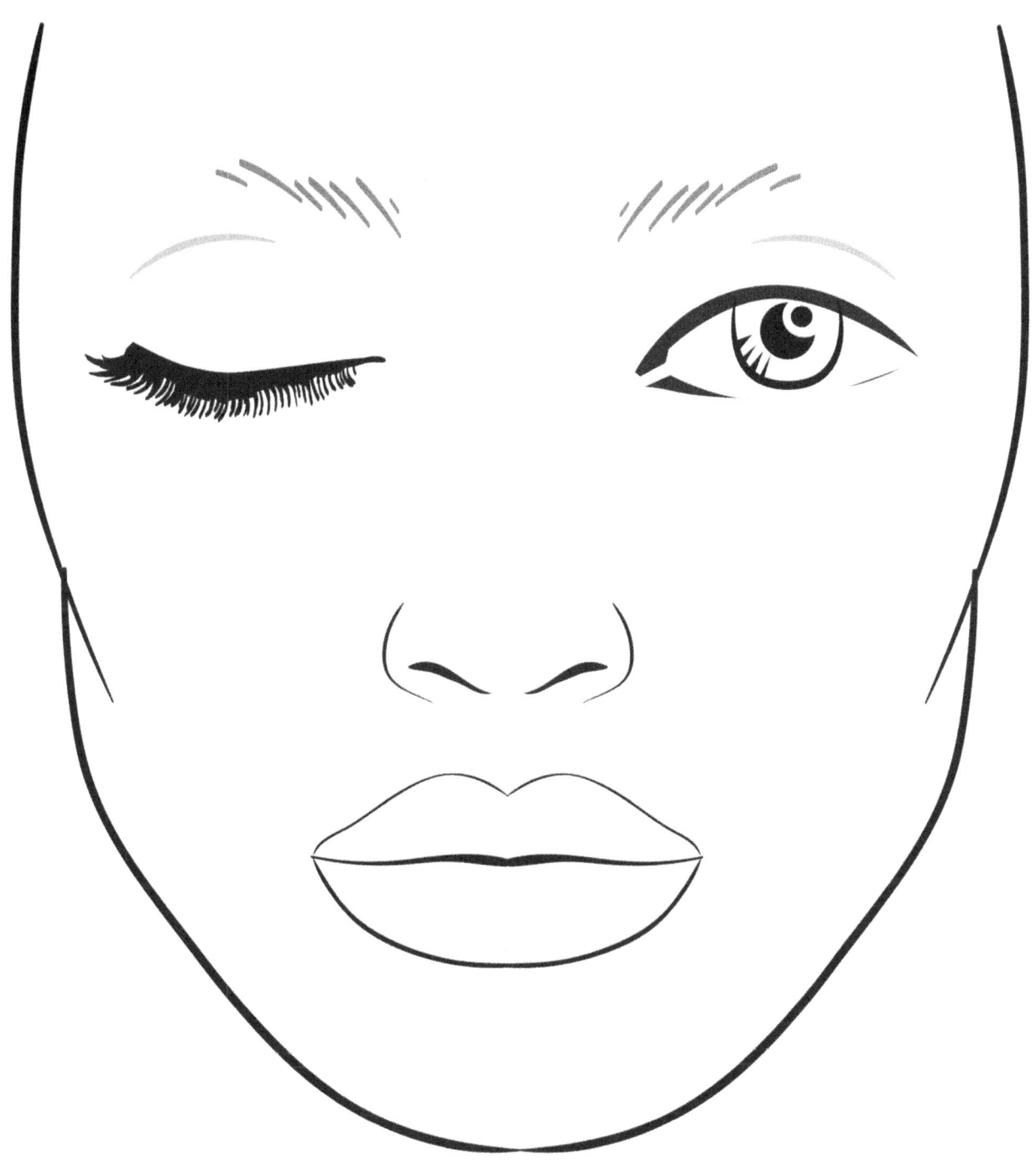

Skin	Eyes	Lips

Client Name: ....
Phone Number: ....
Email Address: ....
Makeup Look: Daytime / Evening / Wedding / Party / Other / (Circle as appropriate).

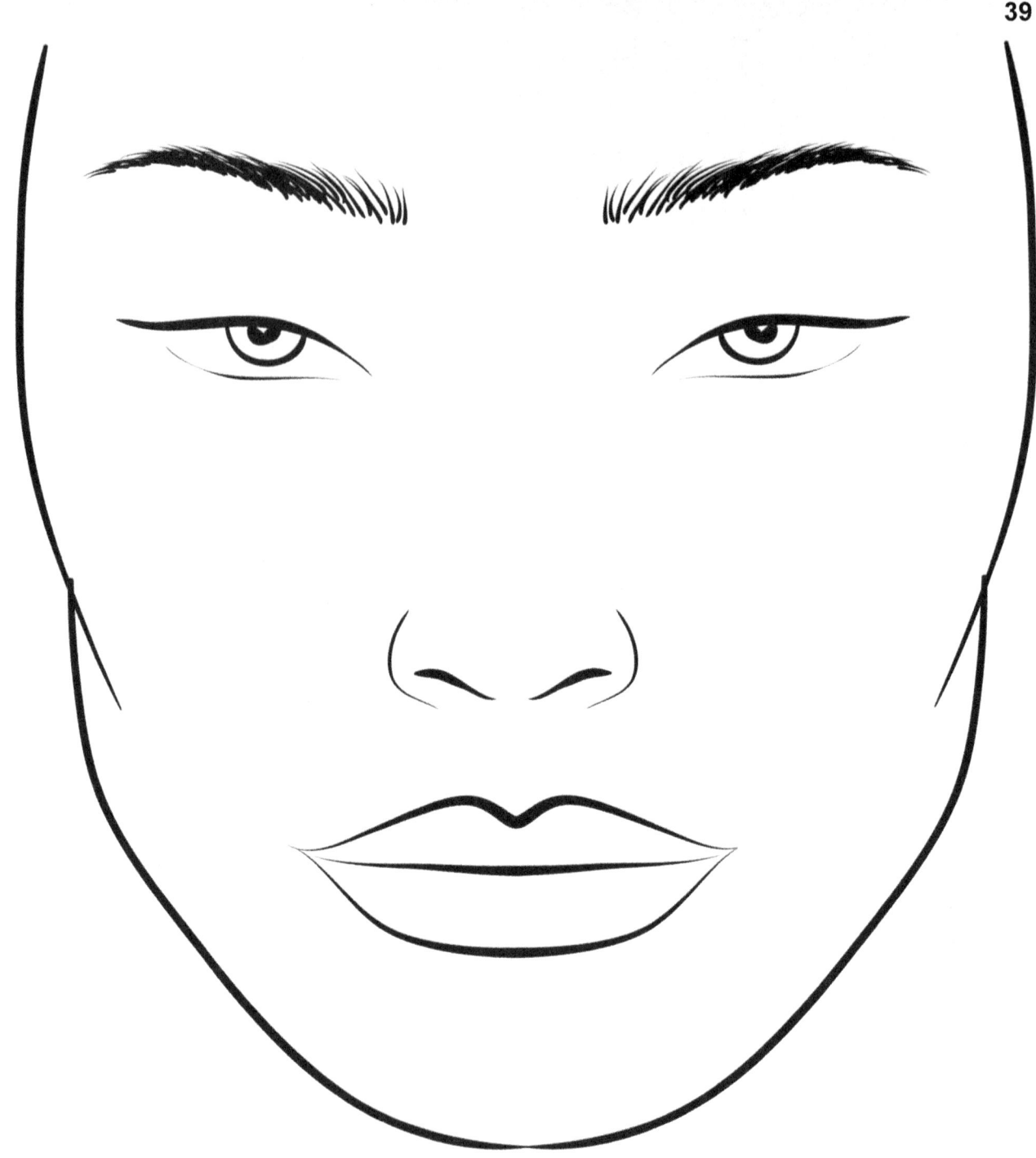

Skin	Eyes	Lips

Client Name: ....
Phone Number: ....
Email Address: ....
Makeup Look: Daytime / Evening / Wedding / Party / Other / (Circle as appropriate).

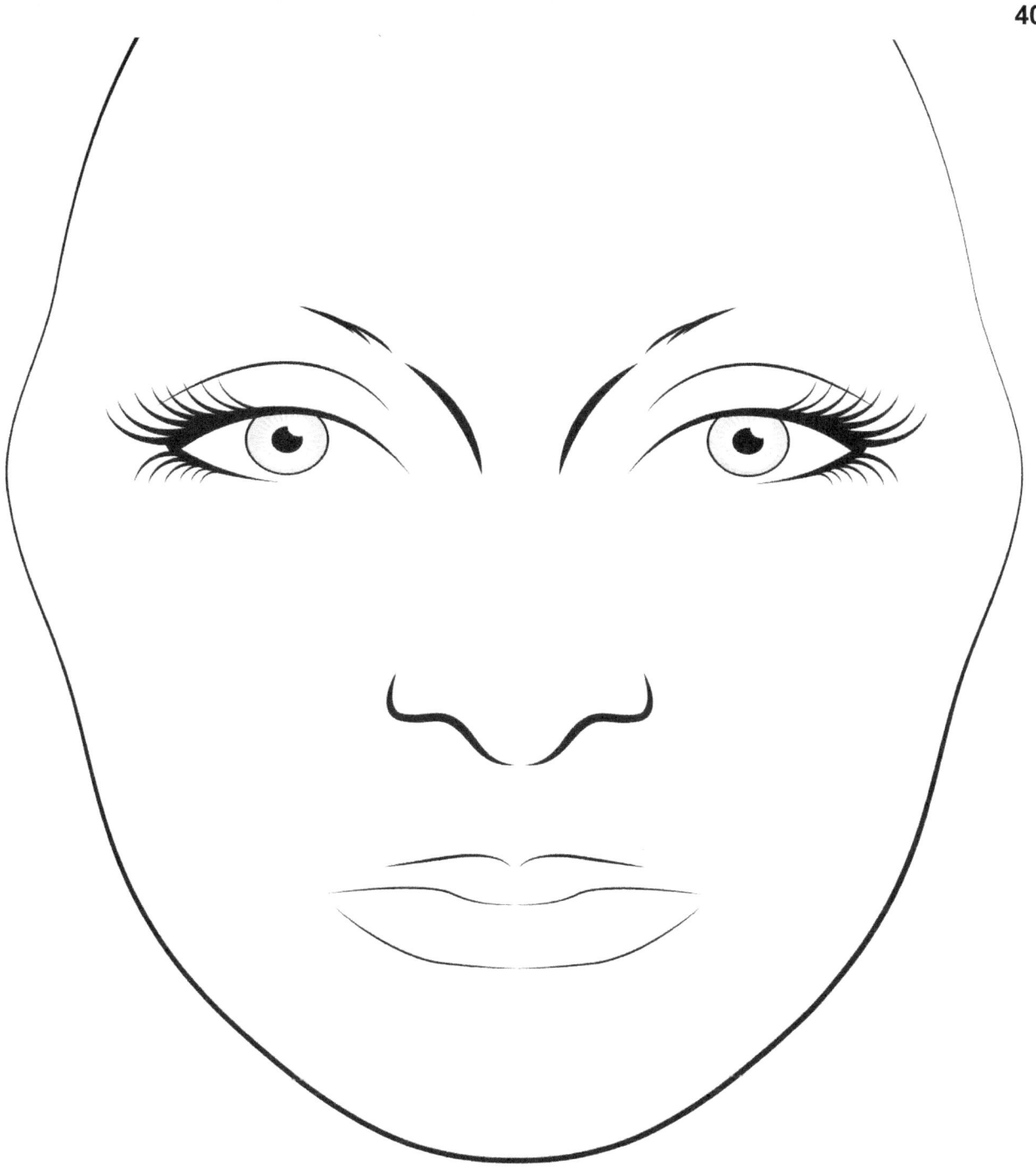

Skin	Eyes	Lips

Client Name: ....
Phone Number: ....
Email Address: ....
Makeup Look: Daytime / Evening / Wedding / Party / Other / (Circle as appropriate).

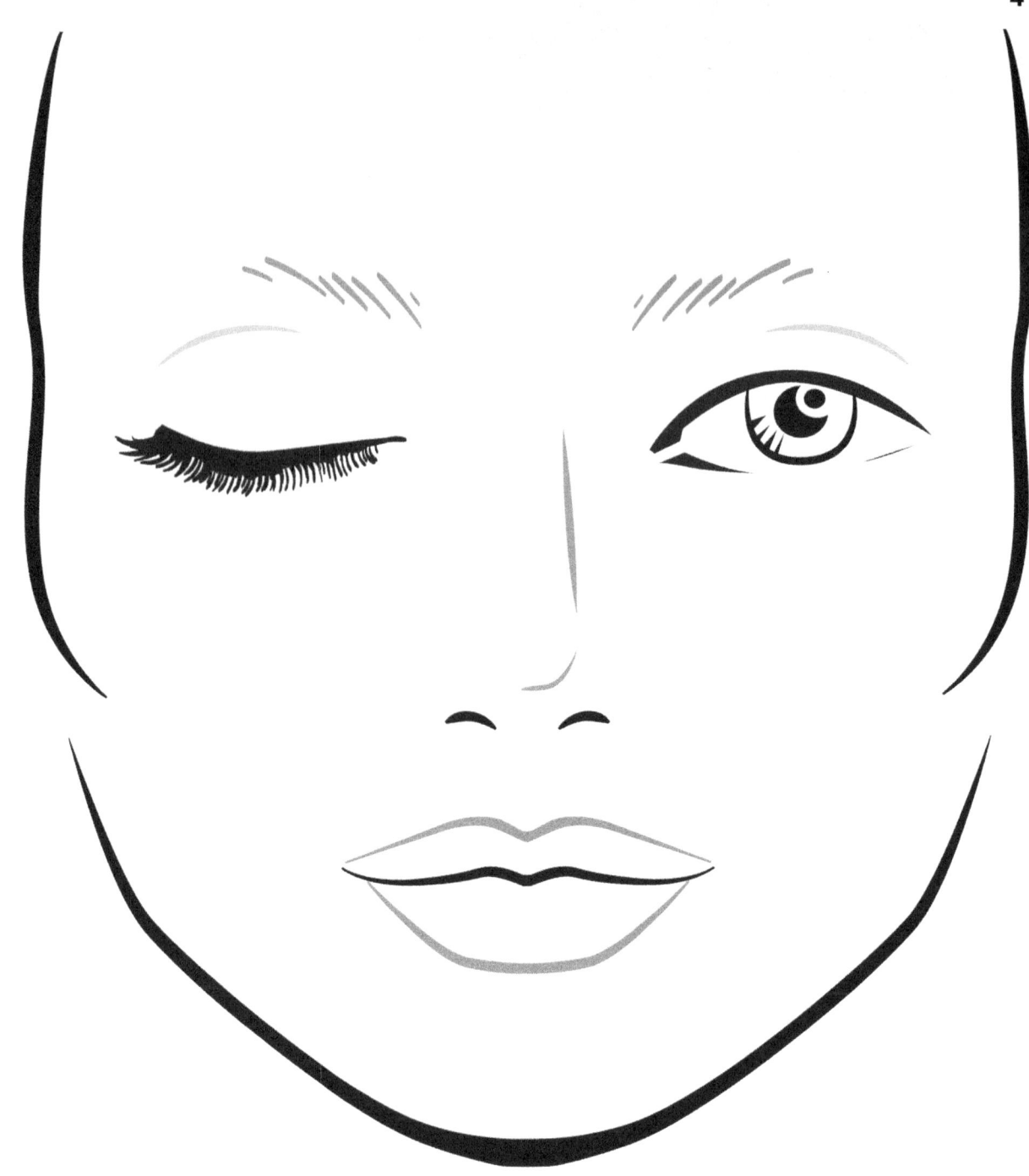

Skin	Eyes	Lips

Client Name: ....

Phone Number: ....

Email Address: ....

Makeup Look: Daytime / Evening / Wedding / Party / Other / (Circle as appropriate).

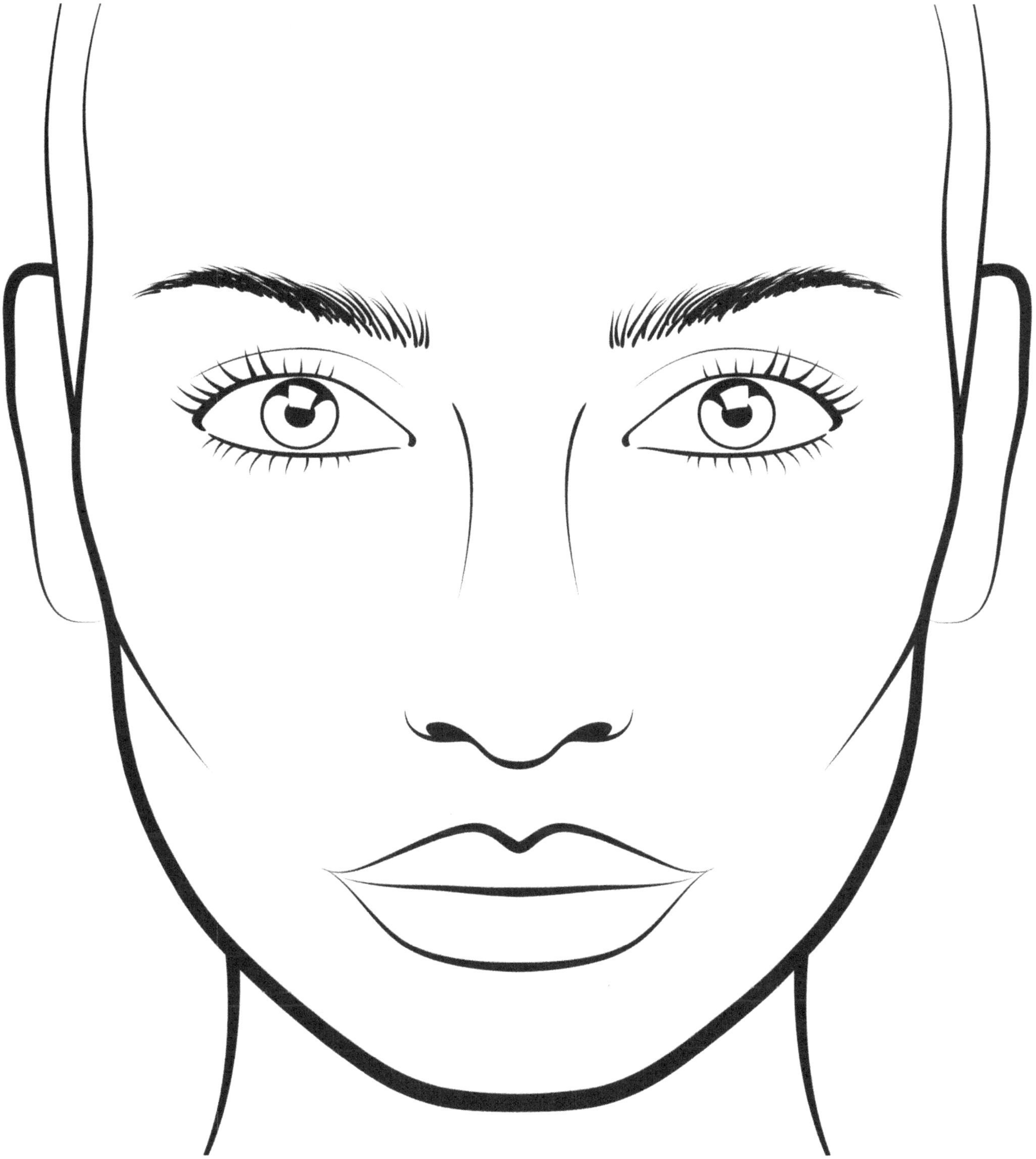

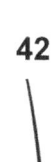

Skin	Eyes	Lips

Client Name: ....
Phone Number: ....
Email Address: ....
Makeup Look: Daytime / Evening / Wedding / Party / Other / (Circle as appropriate).

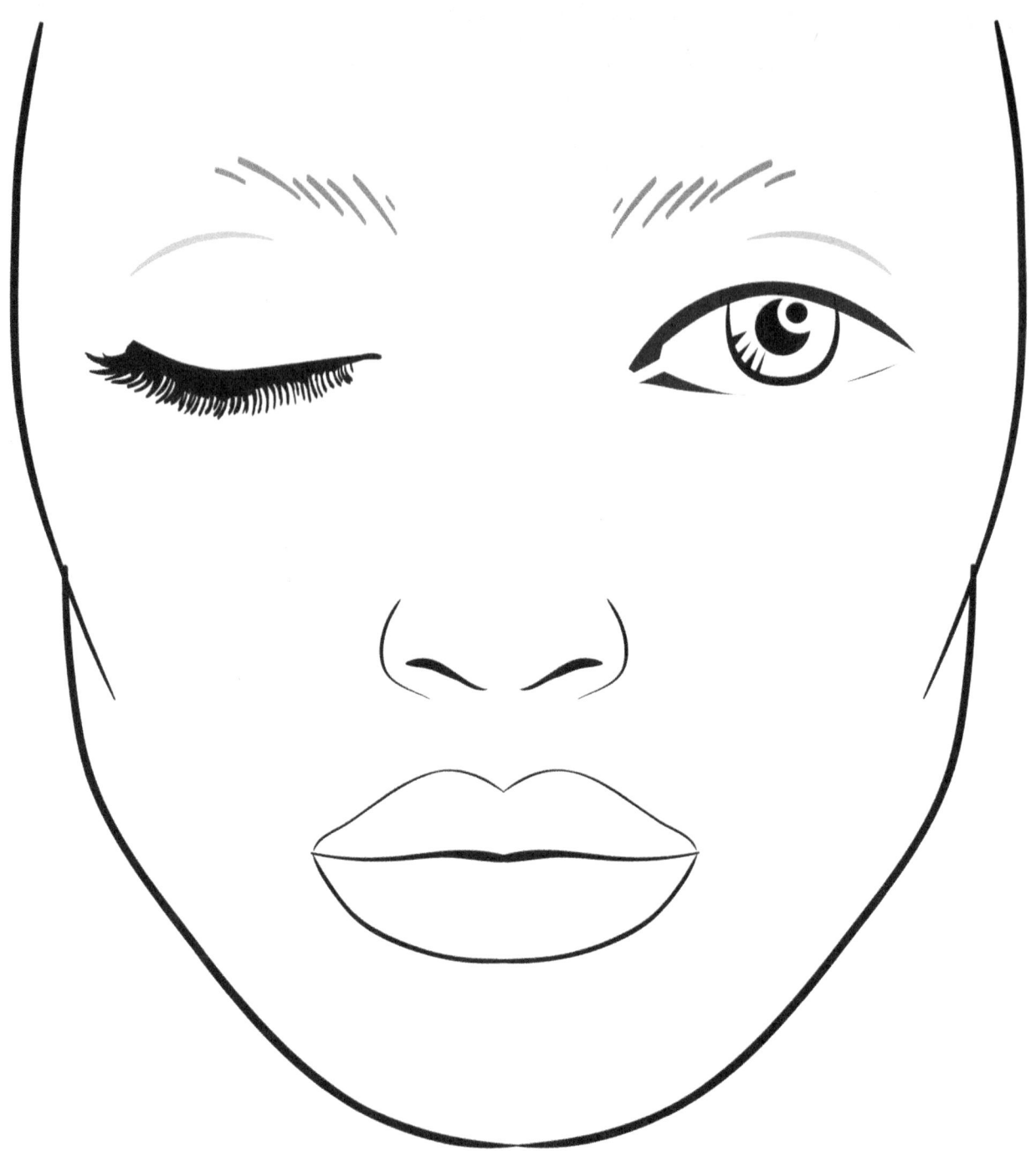

Skin	Eyes	Lips

Client Name: ....
Phone Number: ....
Email Address: ....
Makeup Look: Daytime / Evening / Wedding / Party / Other / (Circle as appropriate).

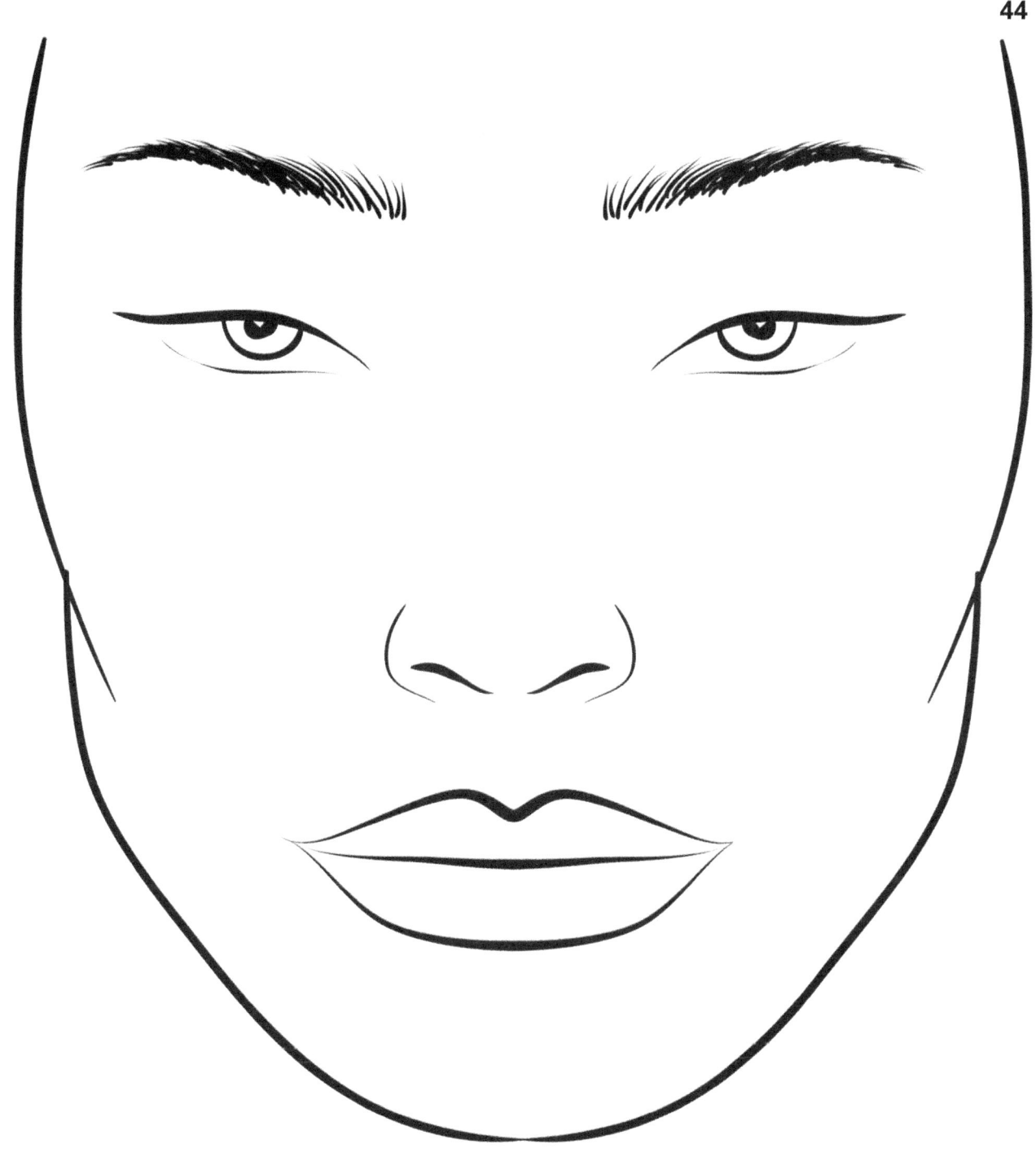

Skin	Eyes	Lips

Client Name: ....
Phone Number: ....
Email Address: ....
Makeup Look: Daytime / Evening / Wedding / Party / Other / (Circle as appropriate).

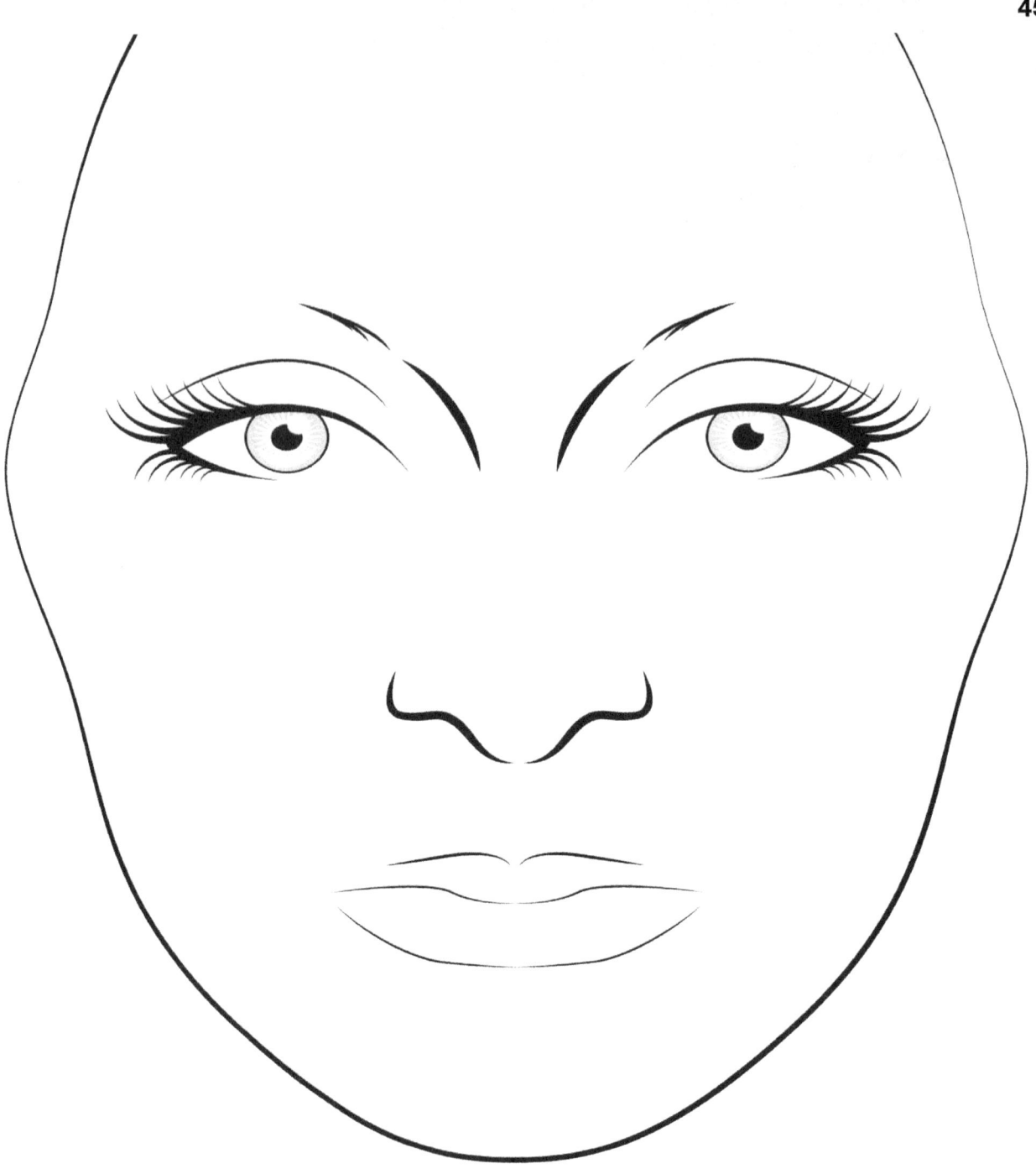

Skin	Eyes	Lips

Client Name: ....
Phone Number: ....
Email Address: ....
Makeup Look: Daytime / Evening / Wedding / Party / Other / (Circle as appropriate).

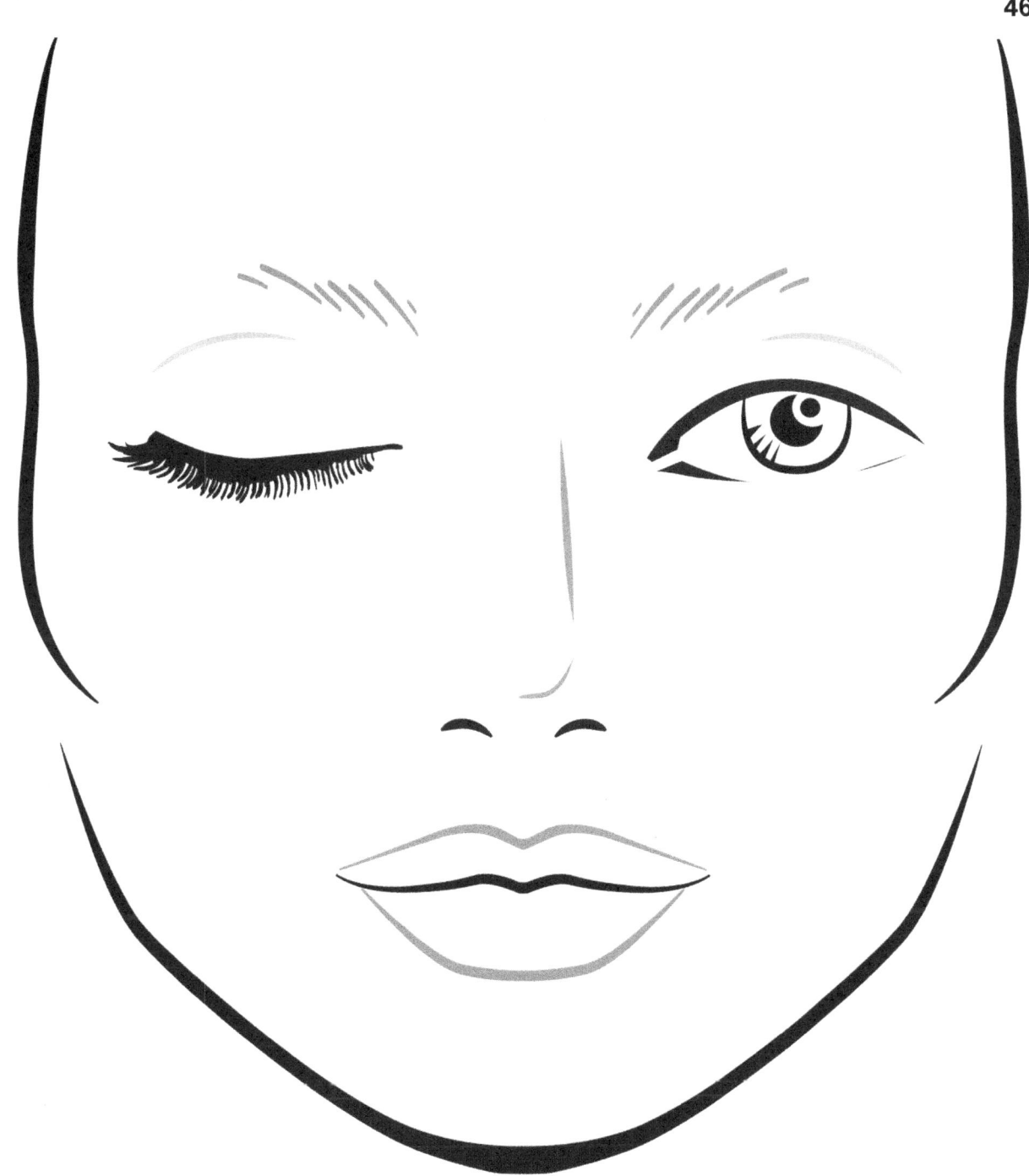

Skin	Eyes	Lips

Client Name: ....

Phone Number: ....

Email Address: ....

Makeup Look: Daytime / Evening / Wedding / Party / Other / (Circle as appropriate).

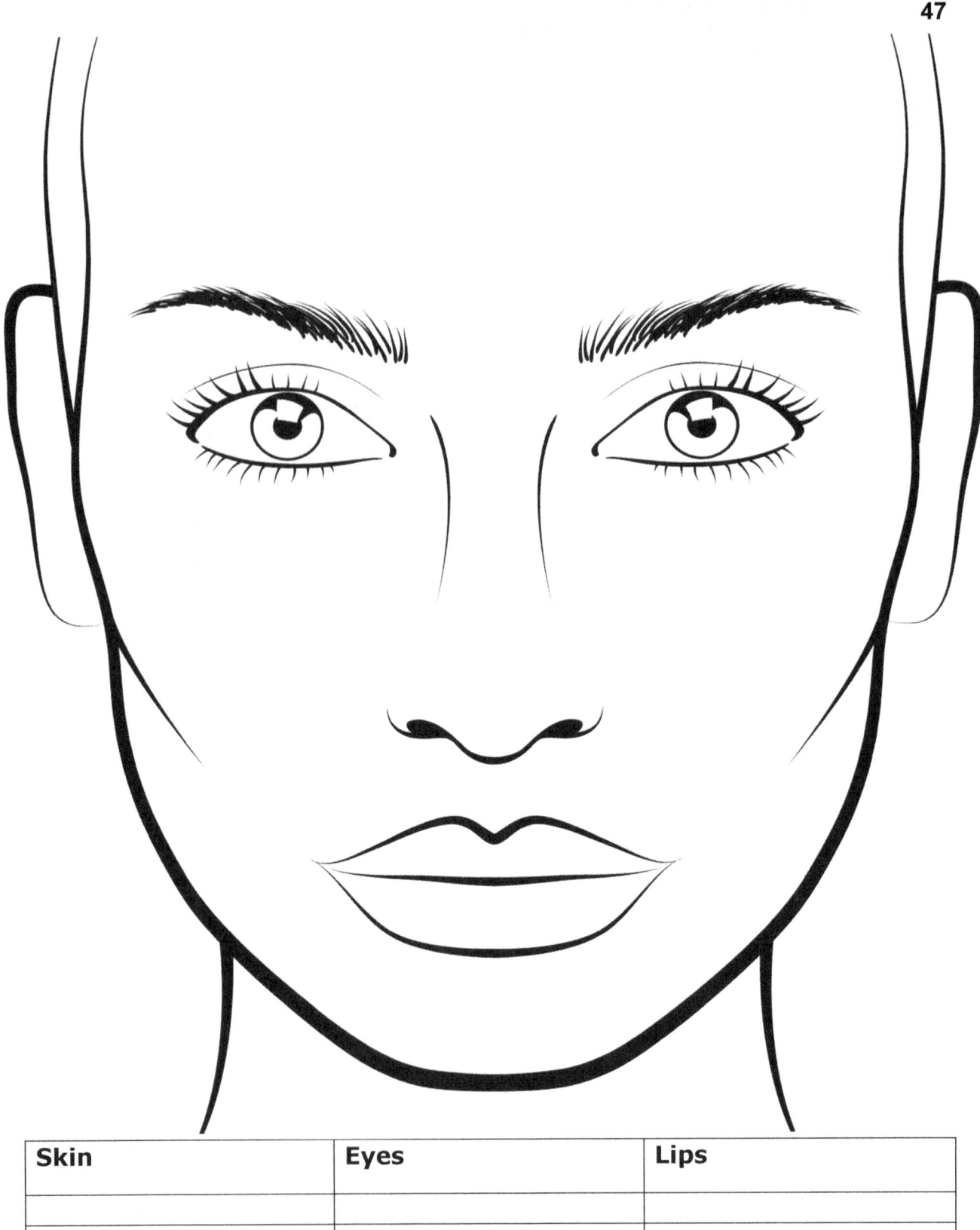

Skin	Eyes	Lips

Client Name: ....
Phone Number: ....
Email Address: ....
Makeup Look: Daytime / Evening / Wedding / Party / Other / (Circle as appropriate).

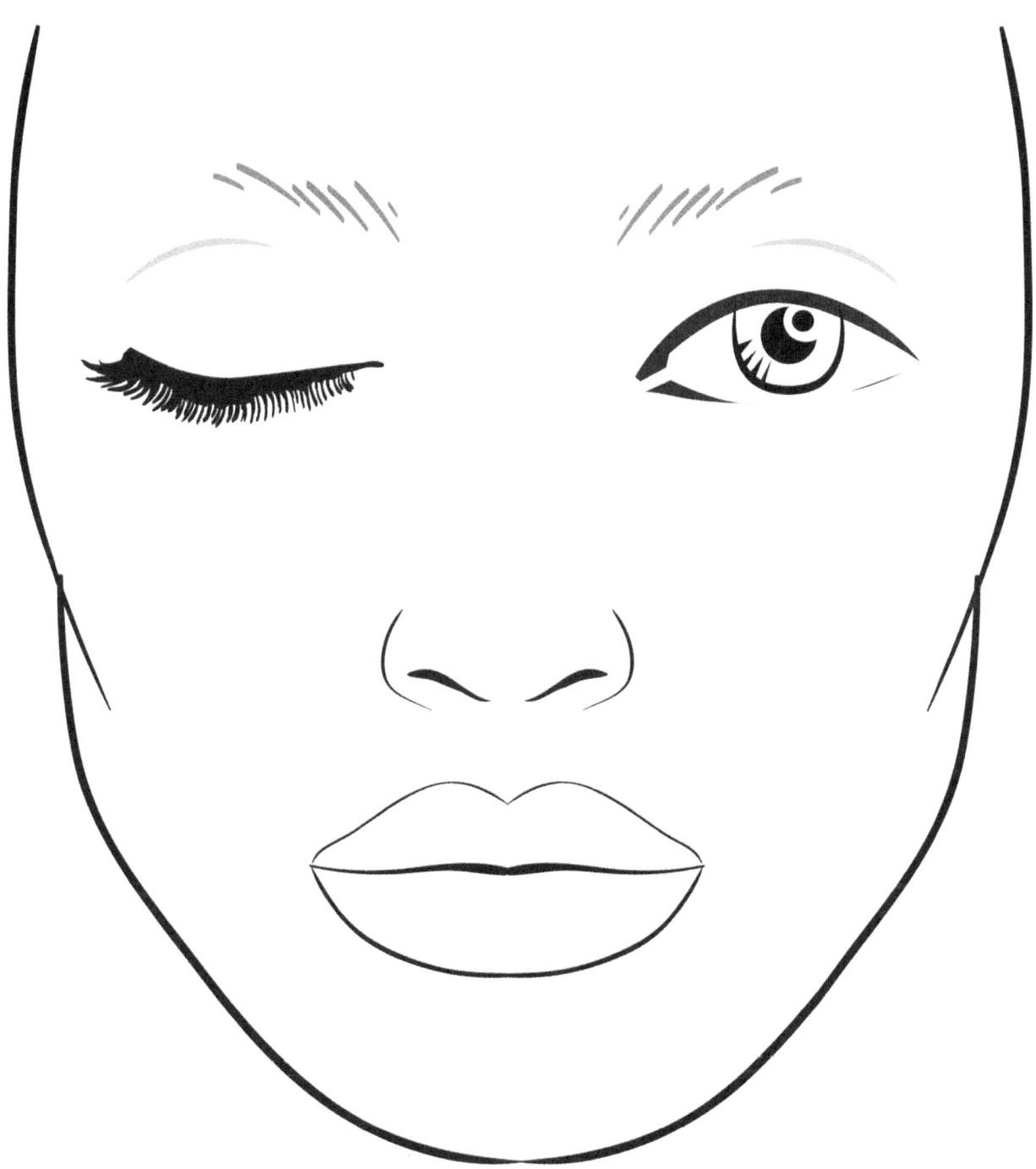

Skin	Eyes	Lips

Client Name: ....
Phone Number: ....
Email Address: ....
Makeup Look: Daytime / Evening / Wedding / Party / Other / (Circle as appropriate).

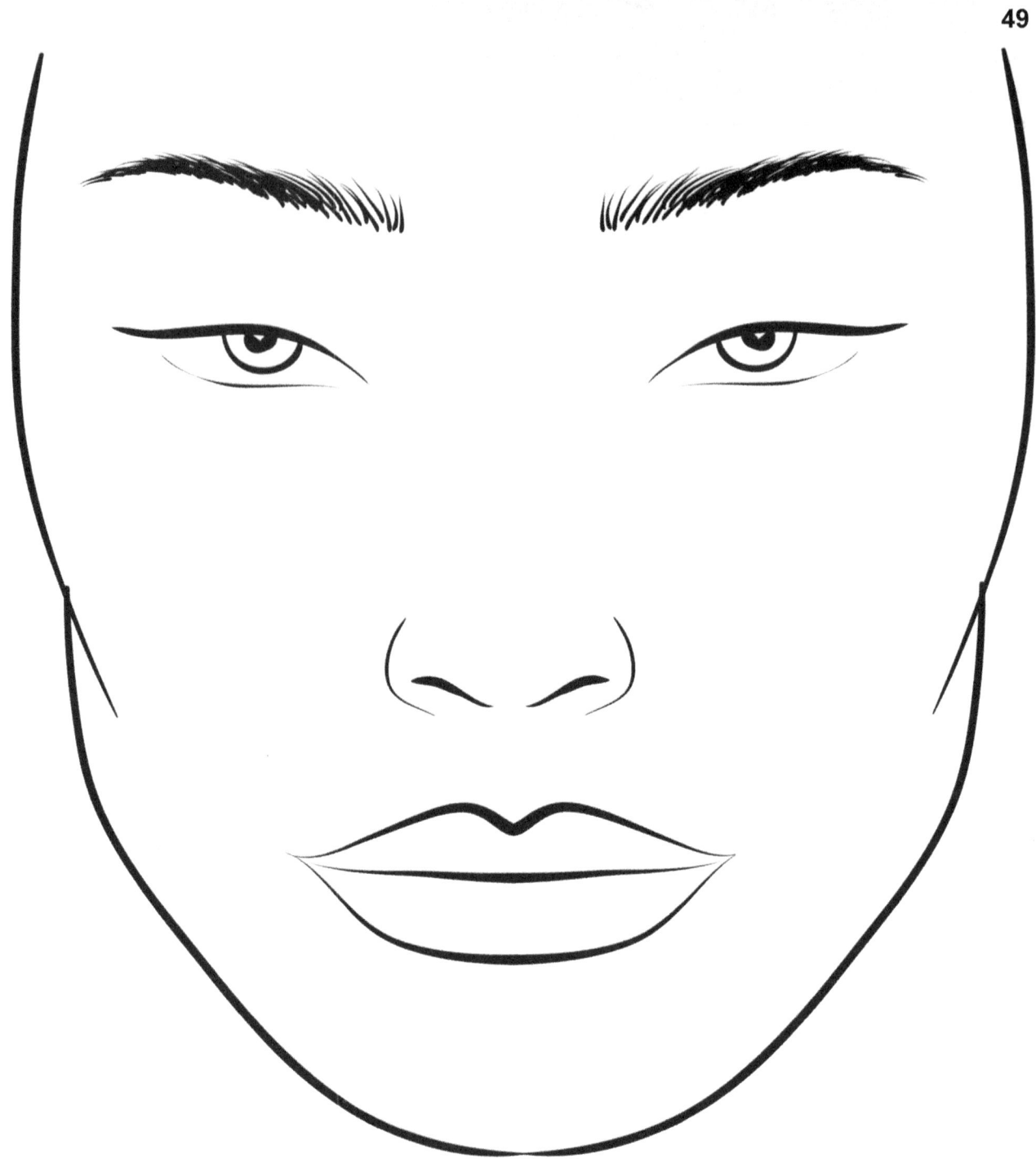

Skin	Eyes	Lips

Client Name: ....
Phone Number: ....
Email Address: ....
Makeup Look: Daytime / Evening / Wedding / Party / Other / (Circle as appropriate).

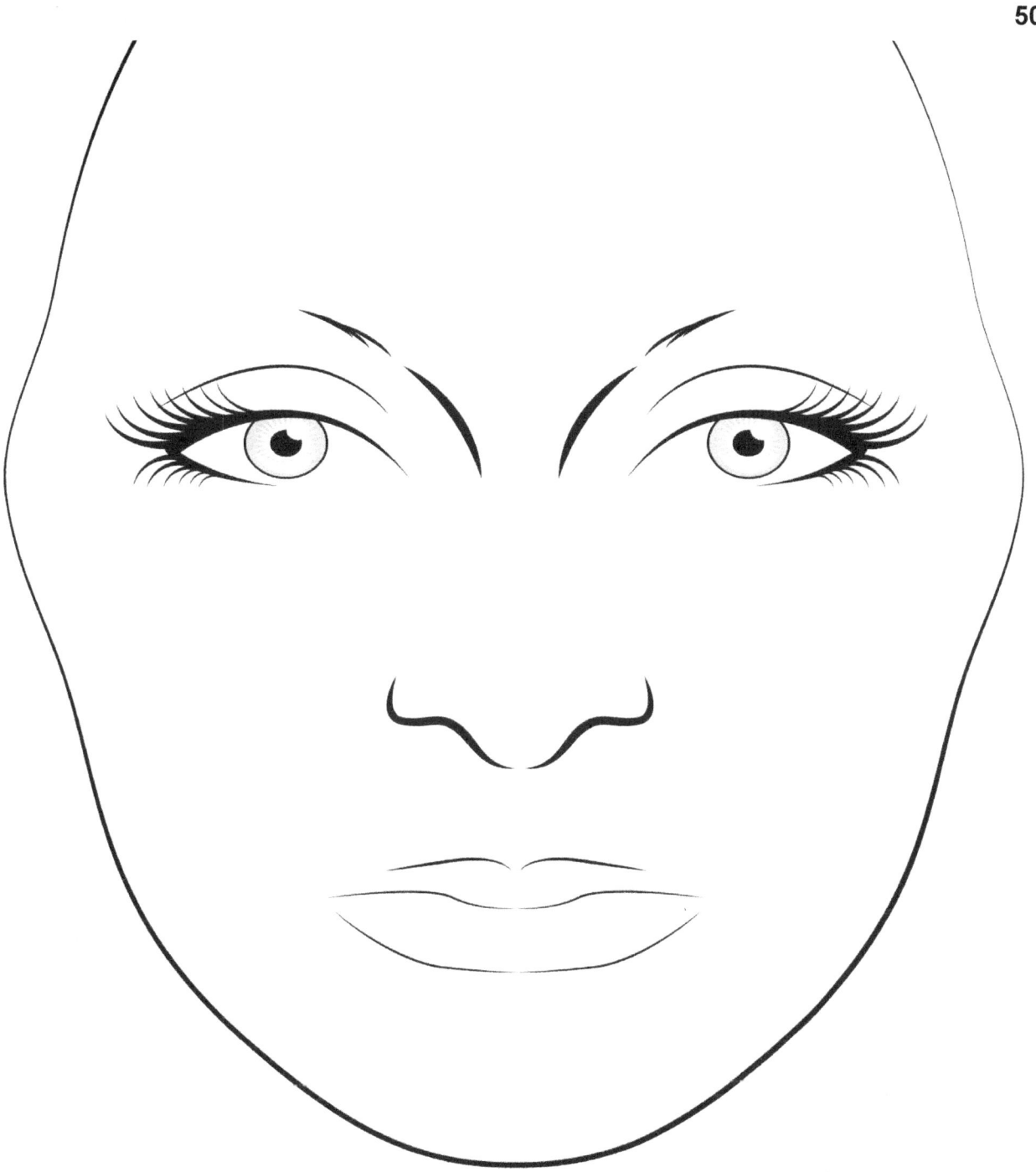

Skin	Eyes	Lips

Client Name: ....
Phone Number: ....
Email Address: ....
Makeup Look: Daytime / Evening / Wedding / Party / Other / (Circle as appropriate).

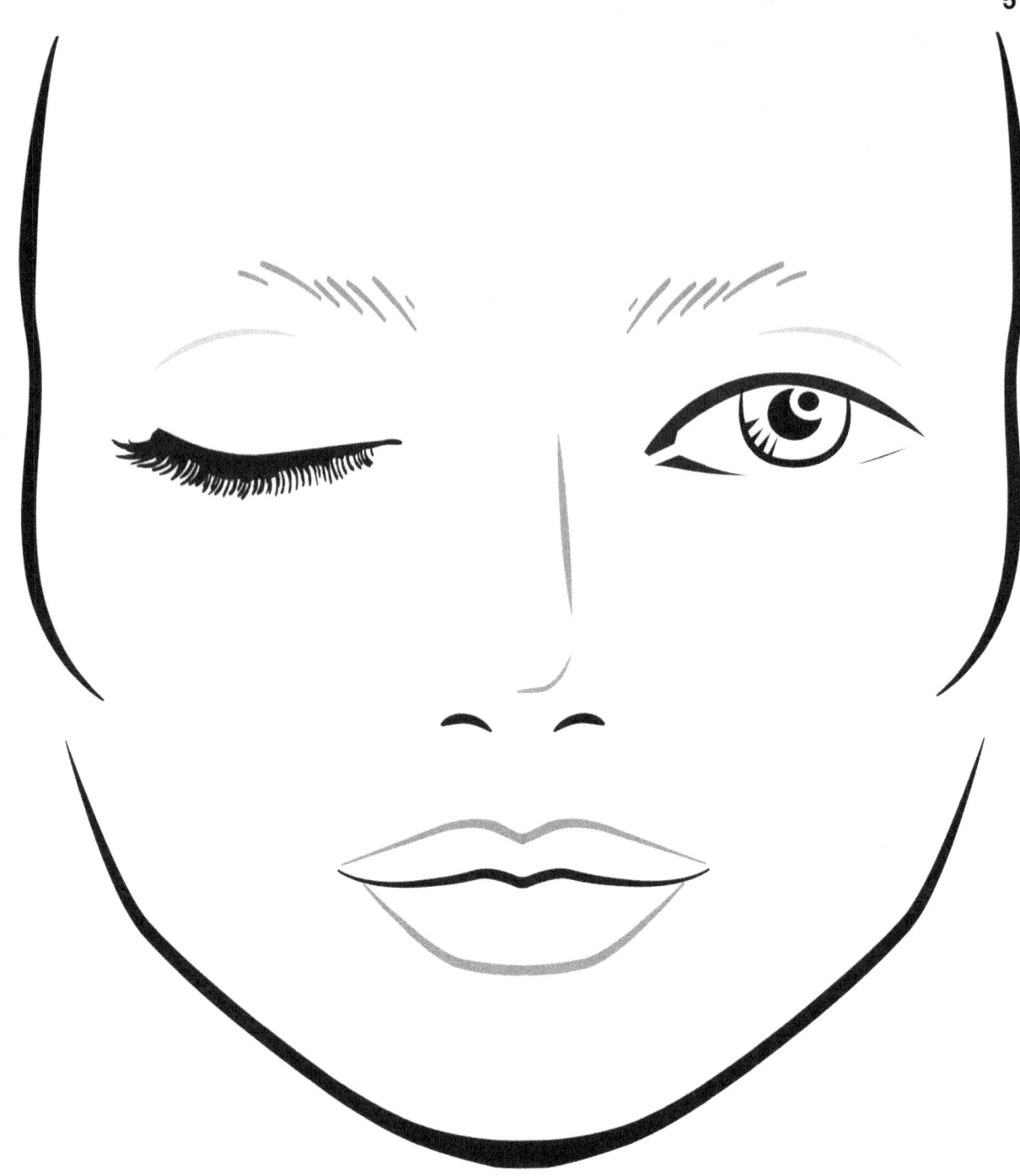

Skin	Eyes	Lips

Client Name: ....
Phone Number: ....
Email Address: ....
Makeup Look: Daytime / Evening / Wedding / Party / Other / (Circle as appropriate).

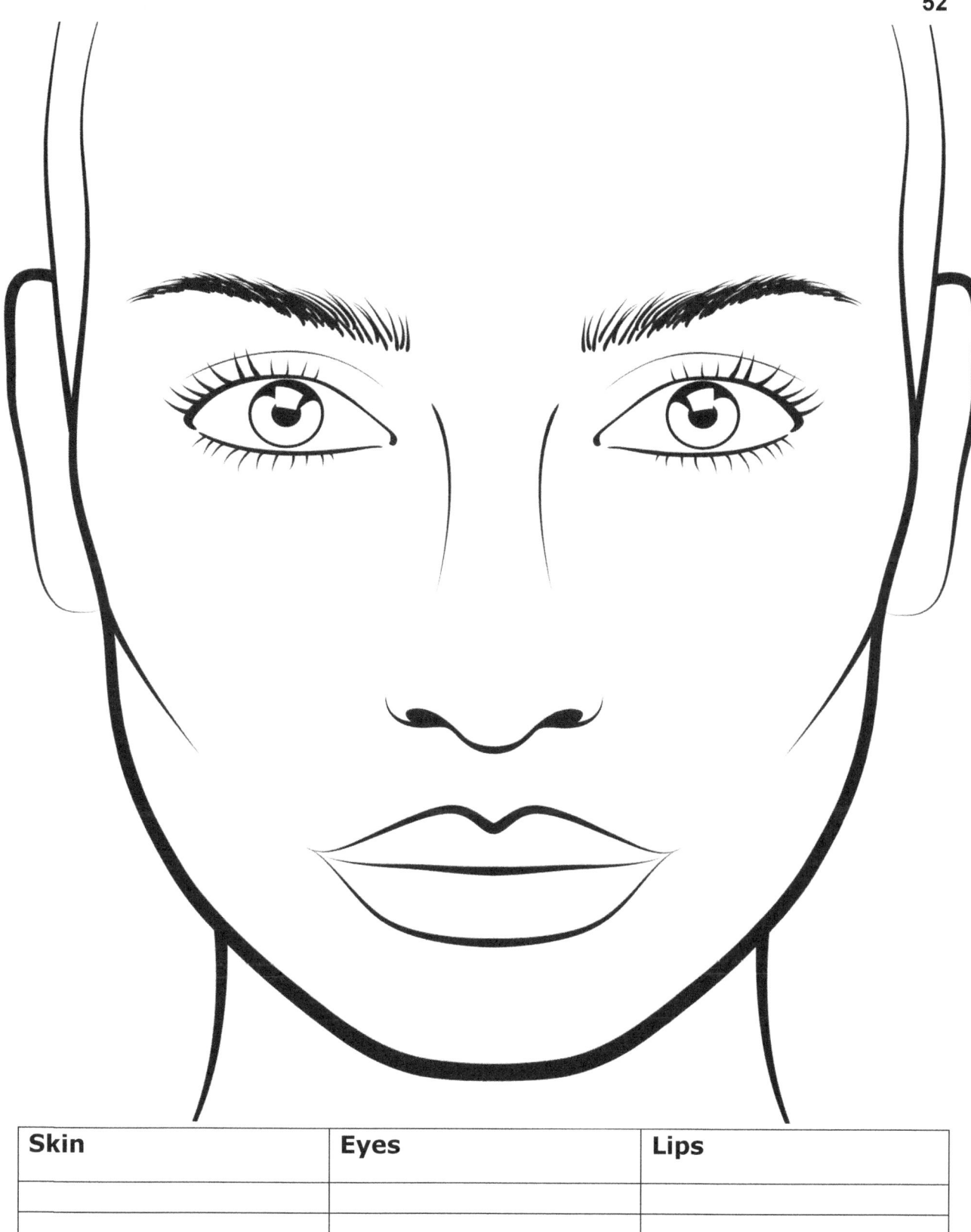

Skin	Eyes	Lips

Client Name: ....
Phone Number: ....
Email Address: ....
Makeup Look: Daytime / Evening / Wedding / Party / Other / (Circle as appropriate).

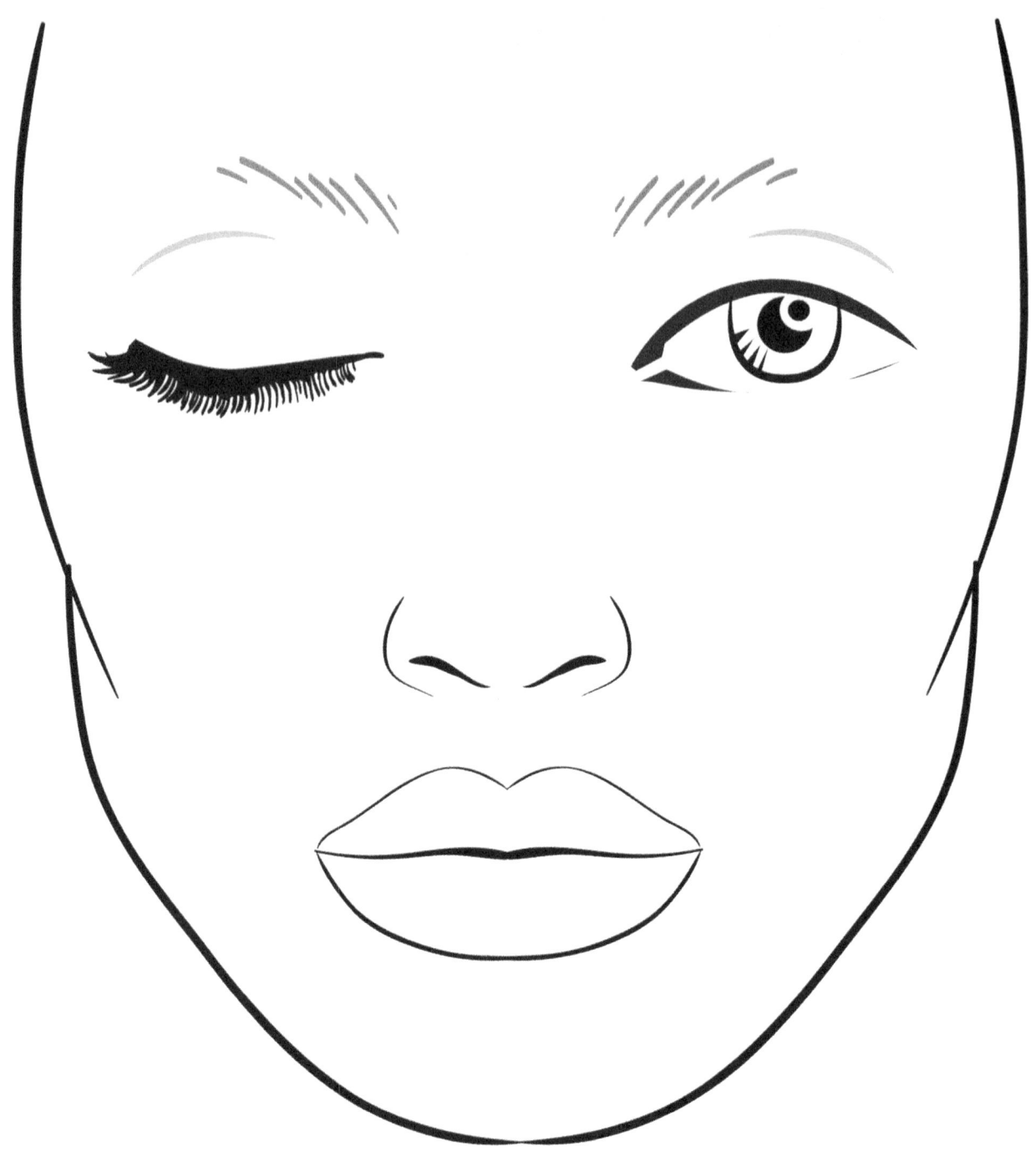

Skin	Eyes	Lips

Client Name: ....

Phone Number: ....

Email Address: ....

Makeup Look: Daytime / Evening / Wedding / Party / Other / (Circle as appropriate).

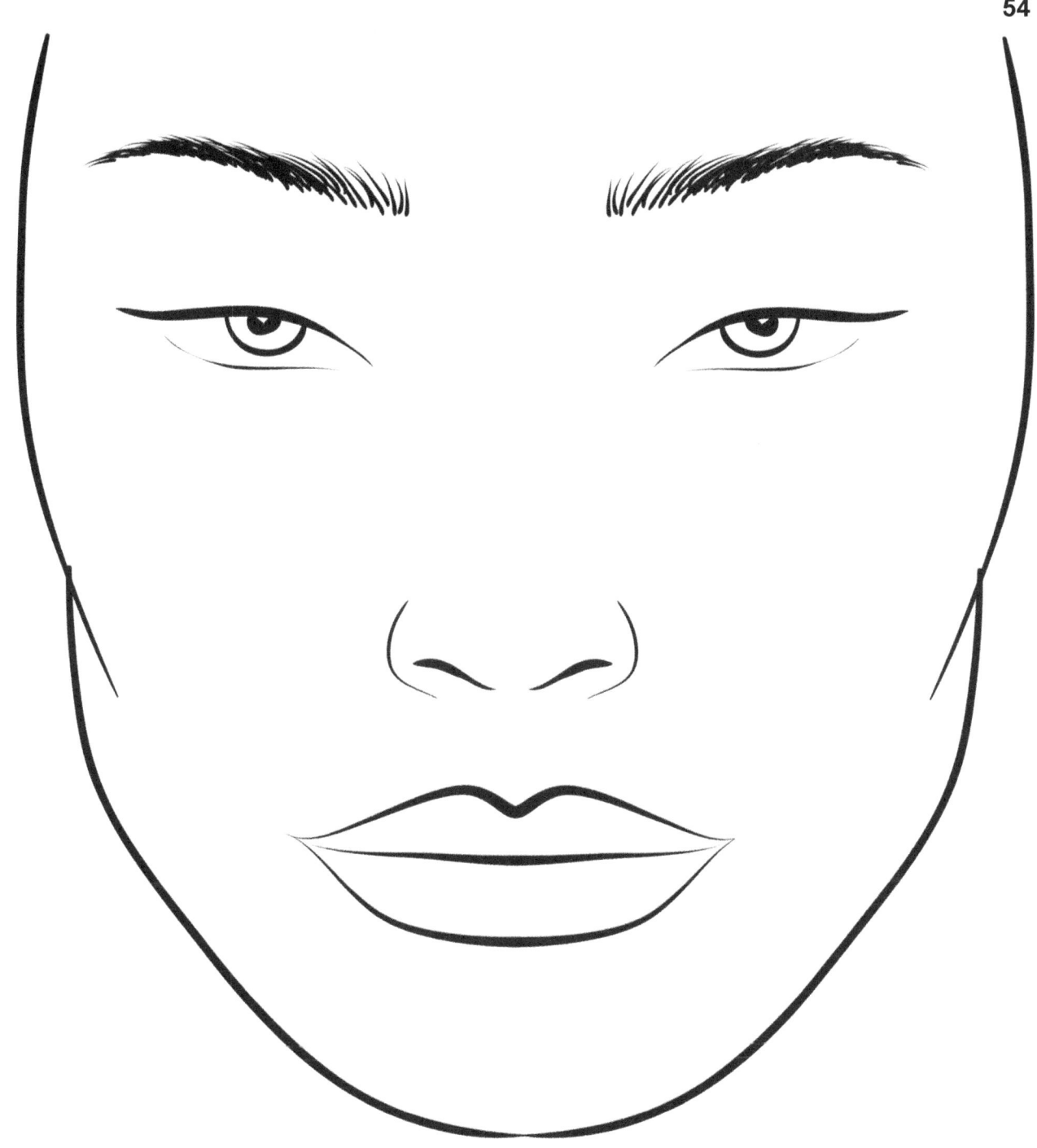

Skin	Eyes	Lips

Client Name: ....
Phone Number: ....
Email Address: ....
Makeup Look: Daytime / Evening / Wedding / Party / Other / (Circle as appropriate).

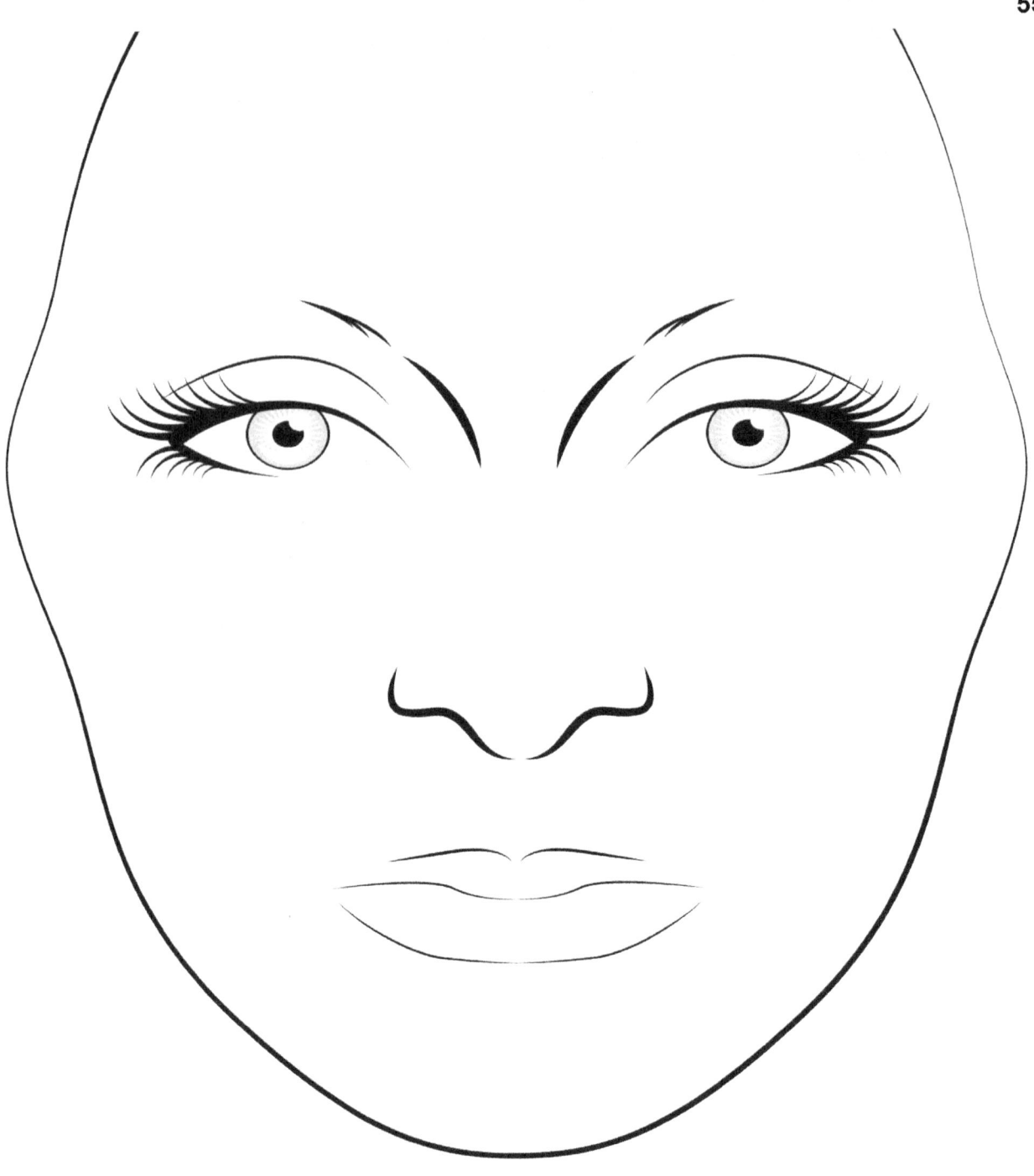

Skin	Eyes	Lips

Client Name: ....
Phone Number: ....
Email Address: ....
Makeup Look: Daytime / Evening / Wedding / Party / Other / (Circle as appropriate).

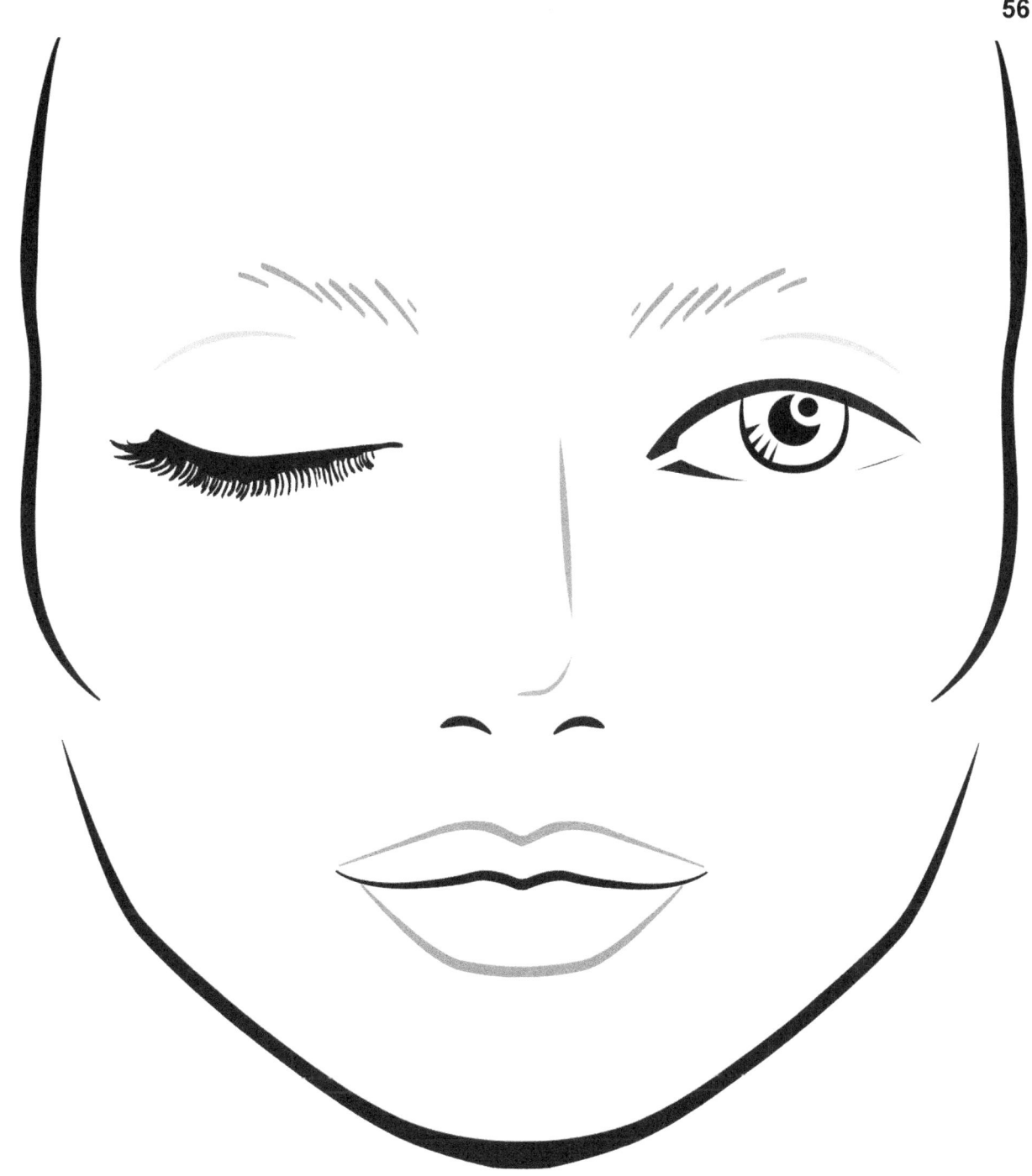

Skin	Eyes	Lips

Client Name: ....
Phone Number: ....
Email Address: ....
Makeup Look: Daytime / Evening / Wedding / Party / Other / (Circle as appropriate).

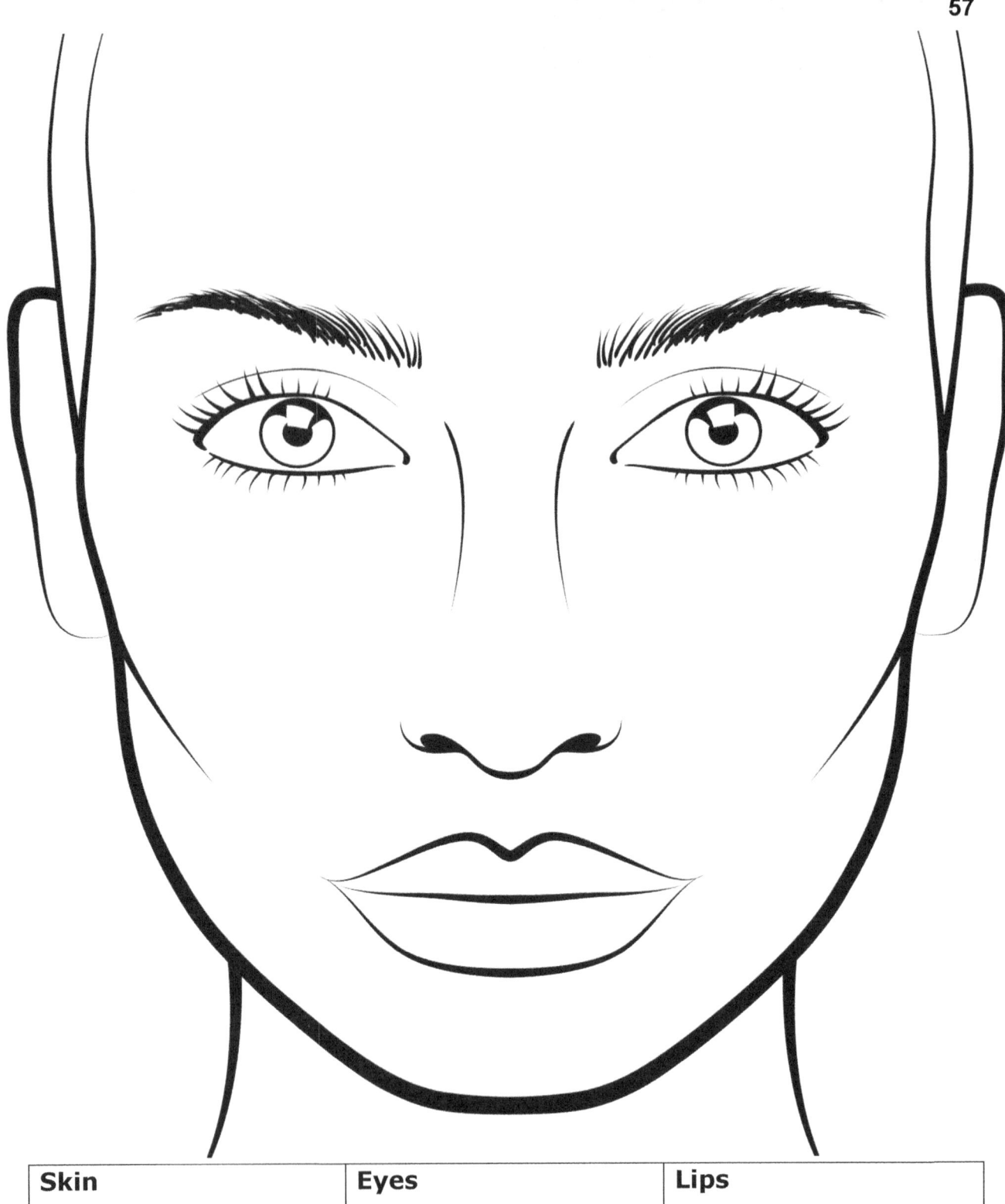

Skin	Eyes	Lips

Client Name: ....
Phone Number: ....
Email Address: ....
Makeup Look: Daytime / Evening / Wedding / Party / Other / (Circle as appropriate).

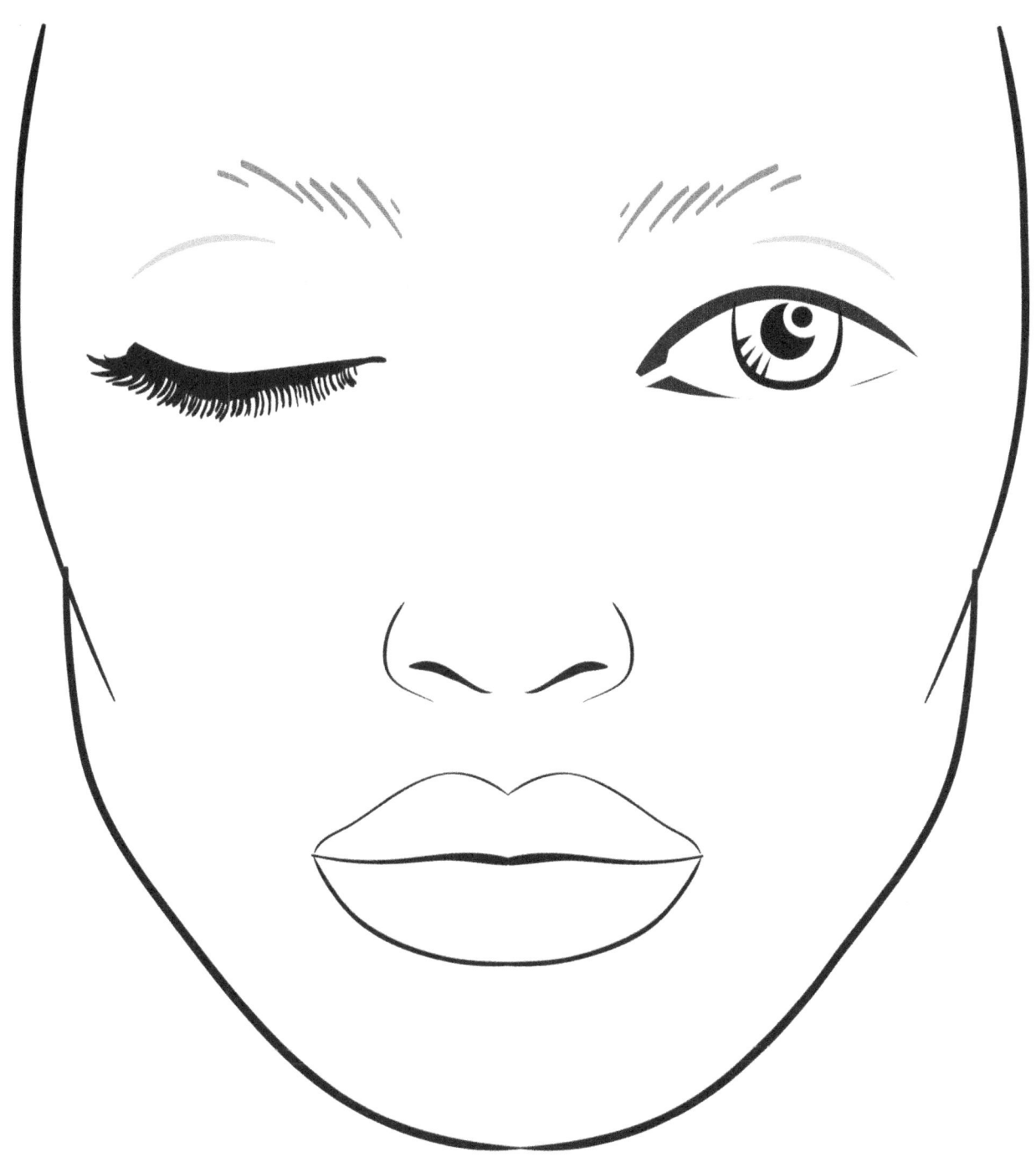

Skin	Eyes	Lips

Client Name: ....
Phone Number: ....
Email Address: ....
Makeup Look: Daytime / Evening / Wedding / Party / Other / (Circle as appropriate).

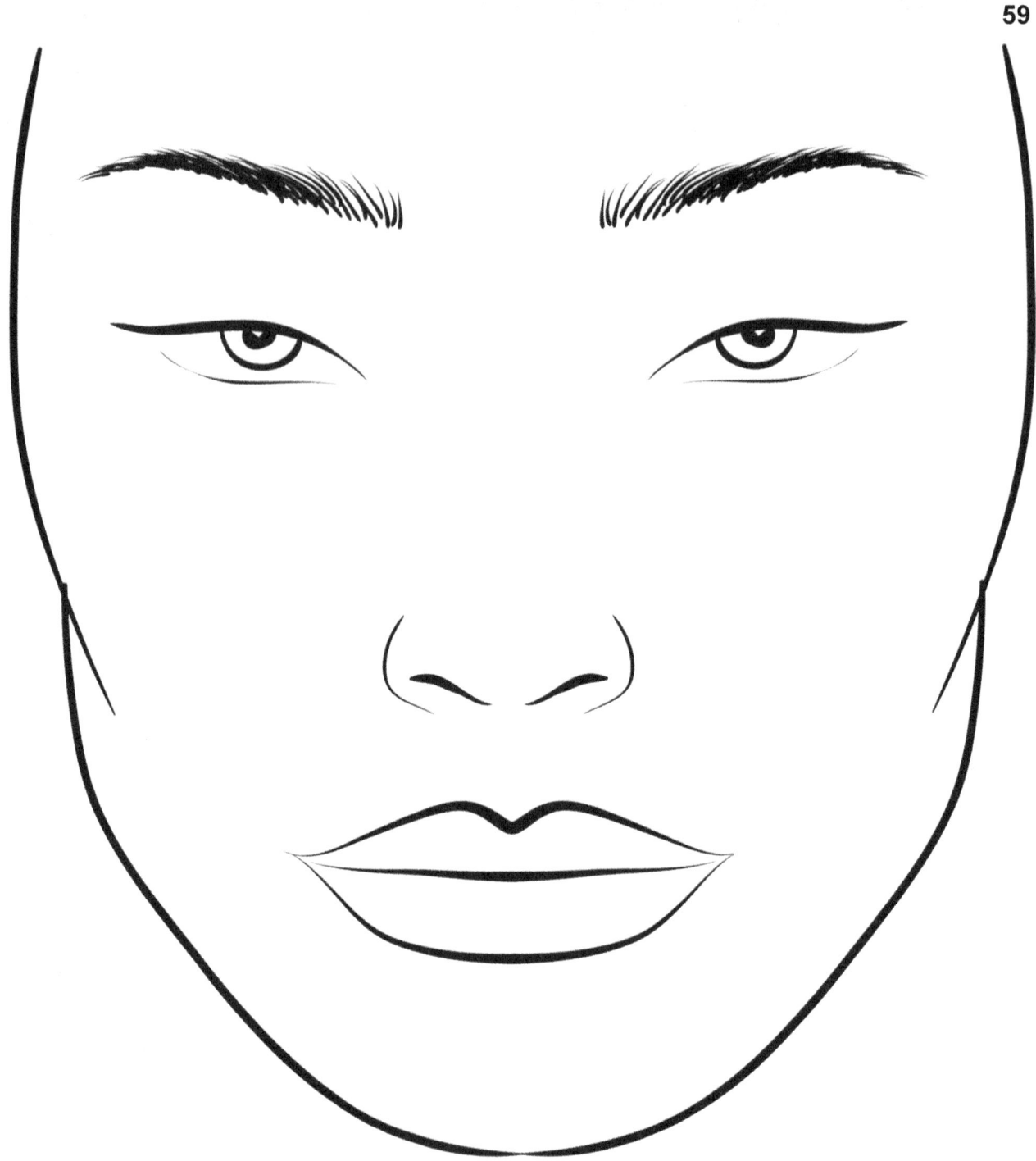

Skin	Eyes	Lips

Client Name: ....
Phone Number: ....
Email Address: ....
Makeup Look: Daytime / Evening / Wedding / Party / Other / (Circle as appropriate).

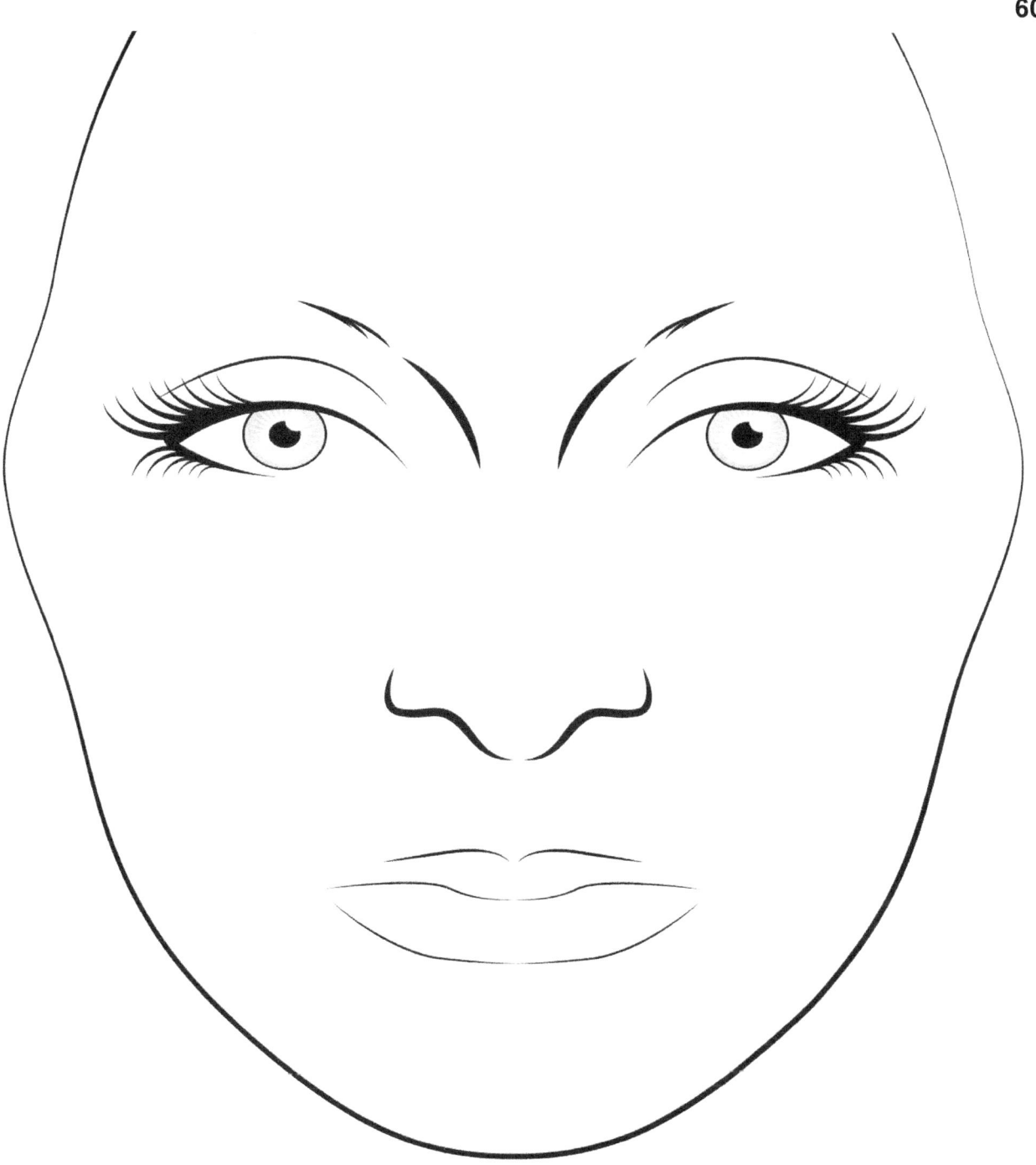

Skin	Eyes	Lips

Client Name: ....

Phone Number: ....

Email Address: ....

Makeup Look: Daytime / Evening / Wedding / Party / Other / (Circle as appropriate).

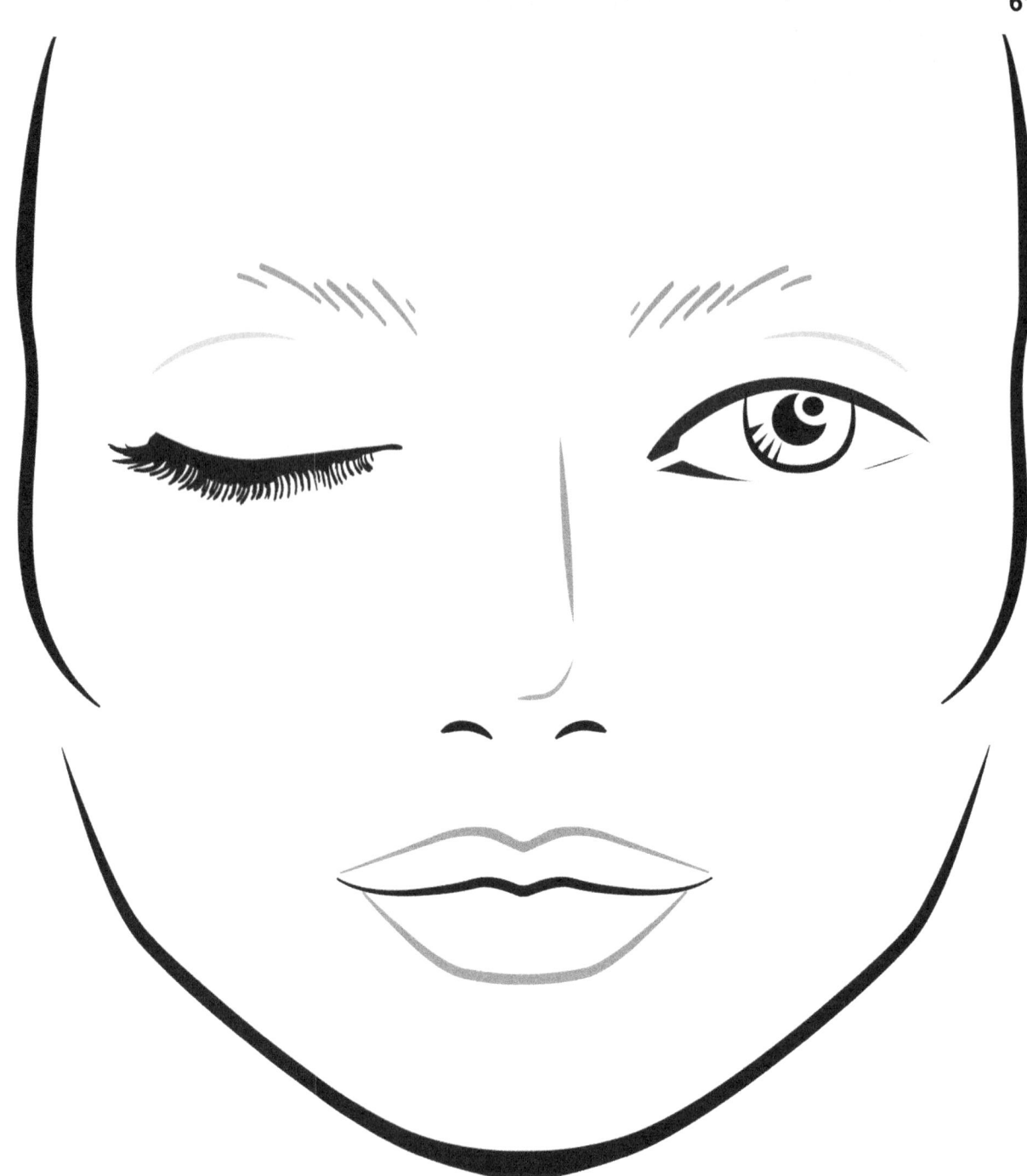

Skin	Eyes	Lips

Client Name: ....
Phone Number: ....
Email Address: ....
Makeup Look: Daytime / Evening / Wedding / Party / Other / (Circle as appropriate).

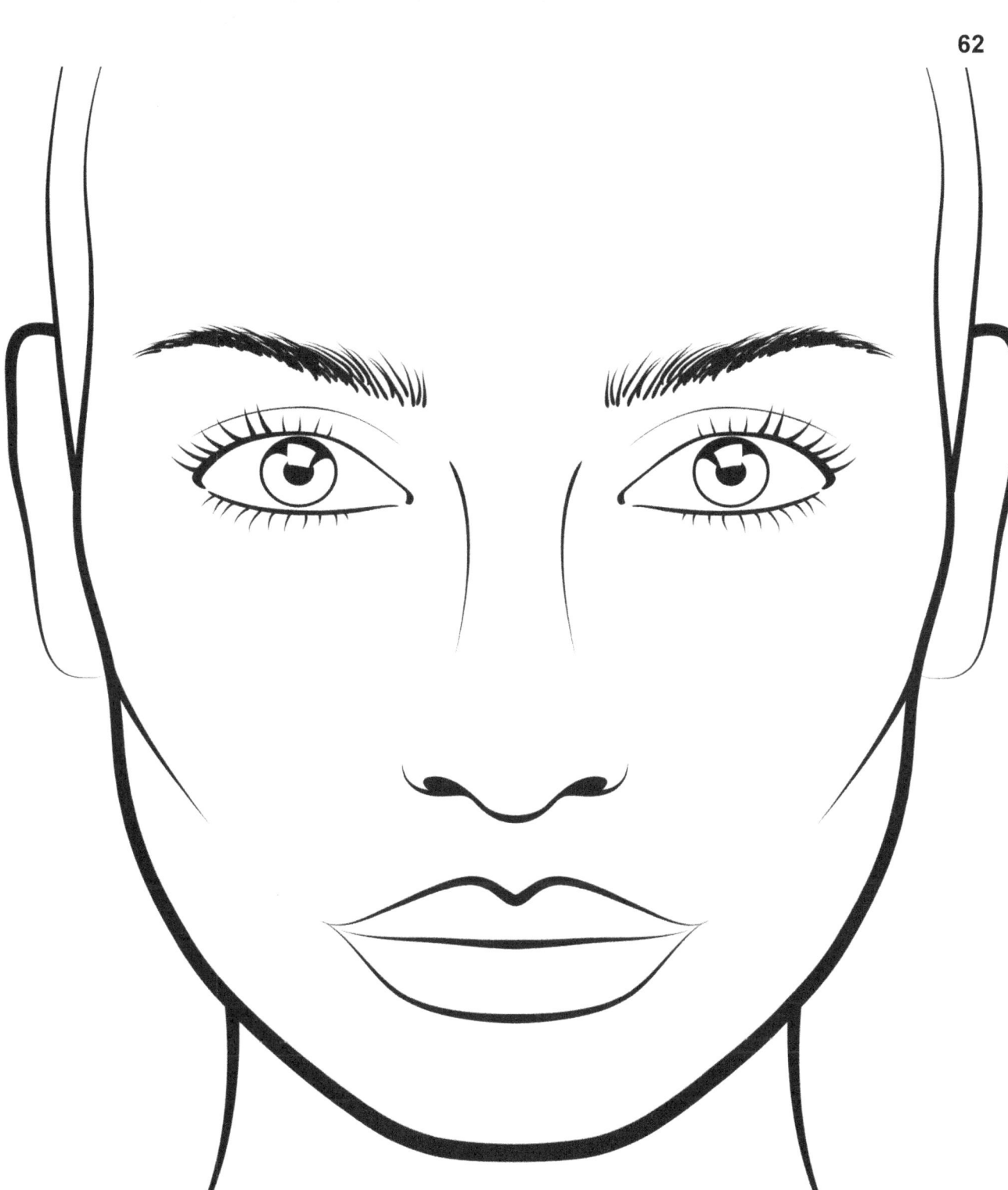

Skin	Eyes	Lips

Client Name: ....
Phone Number: ....
Email Address: ....
Makeup Look: Daytime / Evening / Wedding / Party / Other / (Circle as appropriate).

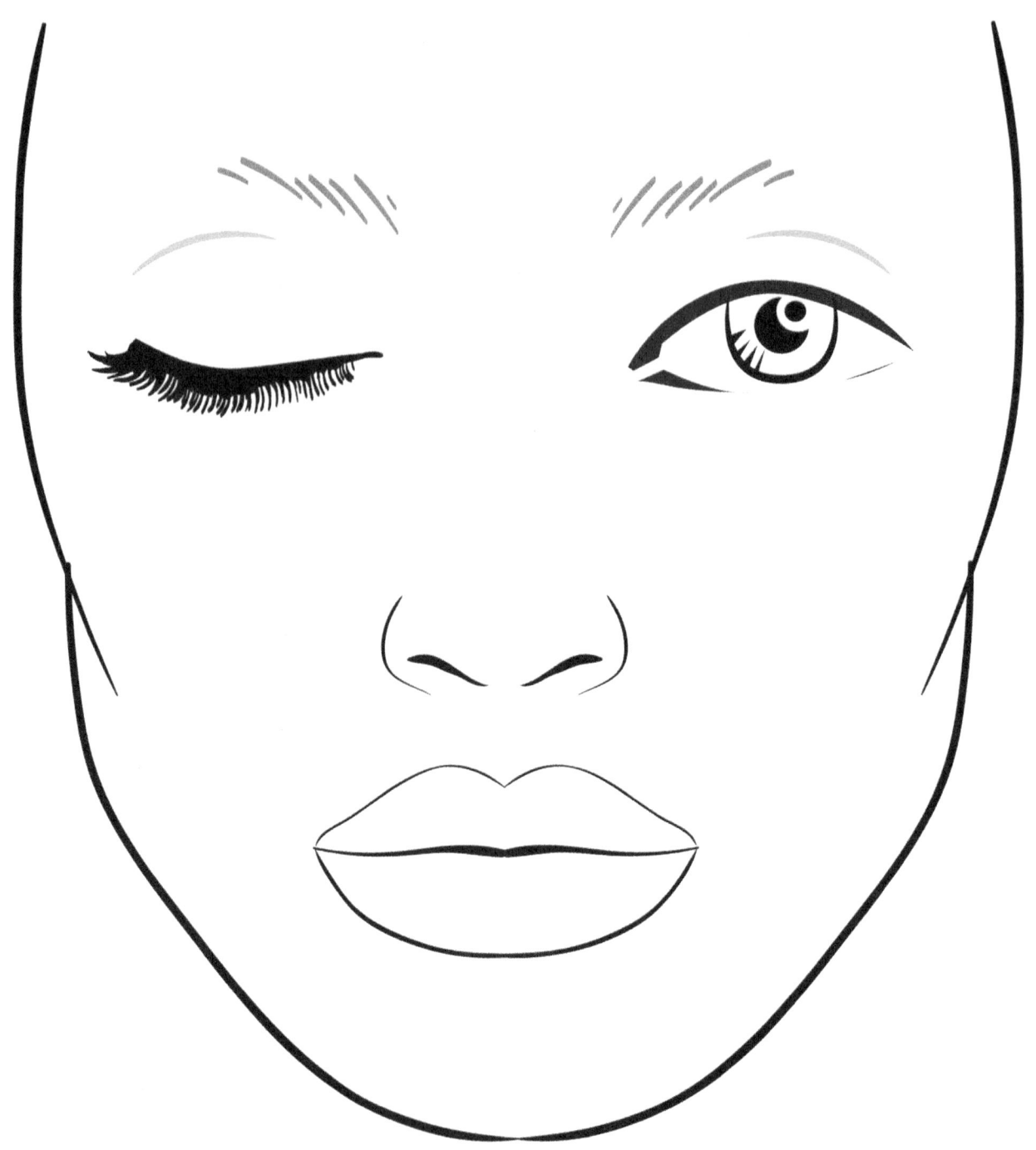

Skin	Eyes	Lips

Client Name: ....
Phone Number: ....
Email Address: ....
Makeup Look: Daytime / Evening / Wedding / Party / Other / (Circle as appropriate).

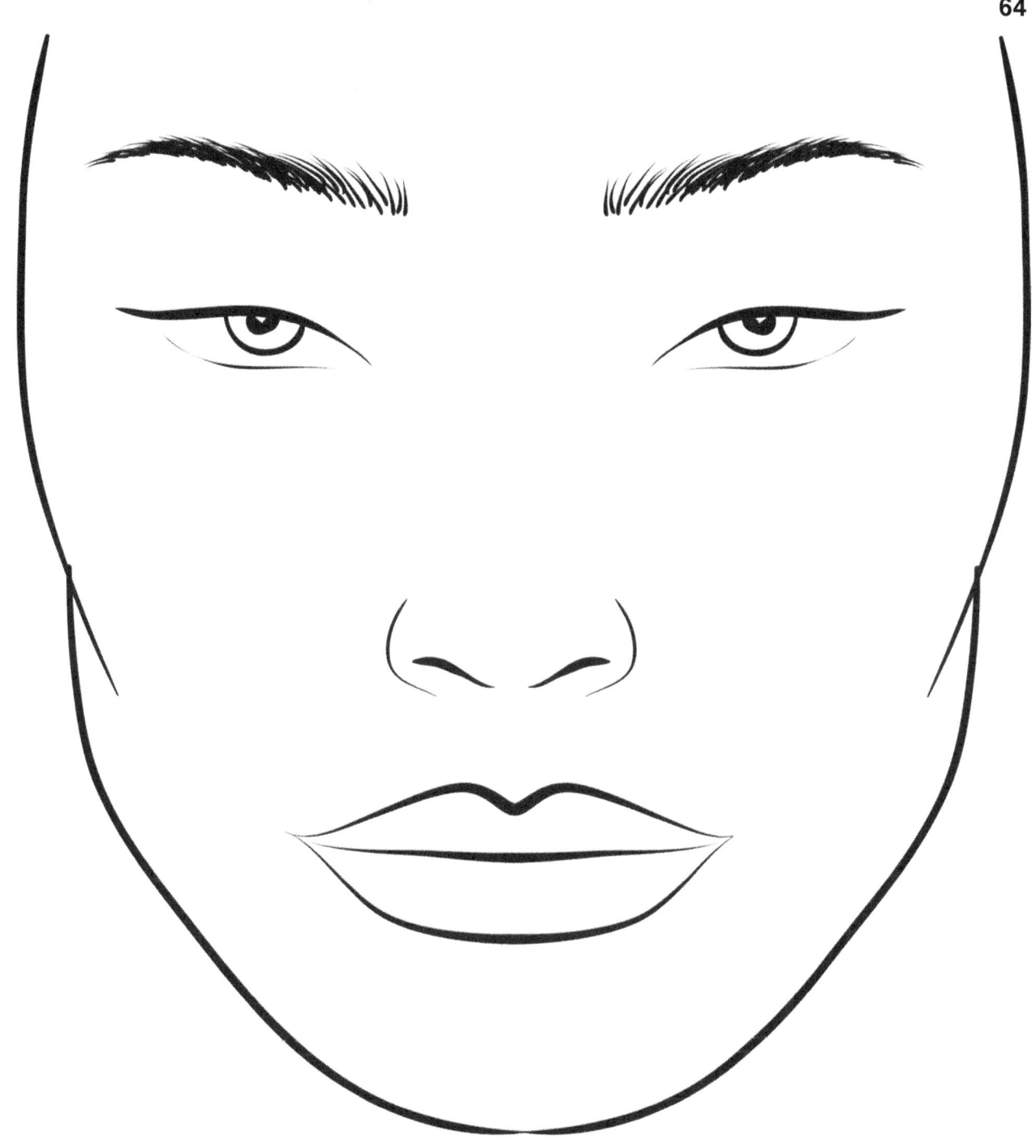

Skin	Eyes	Lips

Client Name: ....
Phone Number: ....
Email Address: ....
Makeup Look: Daytime / Evening / Wedding / Party / Other / (Circle as appropriate).

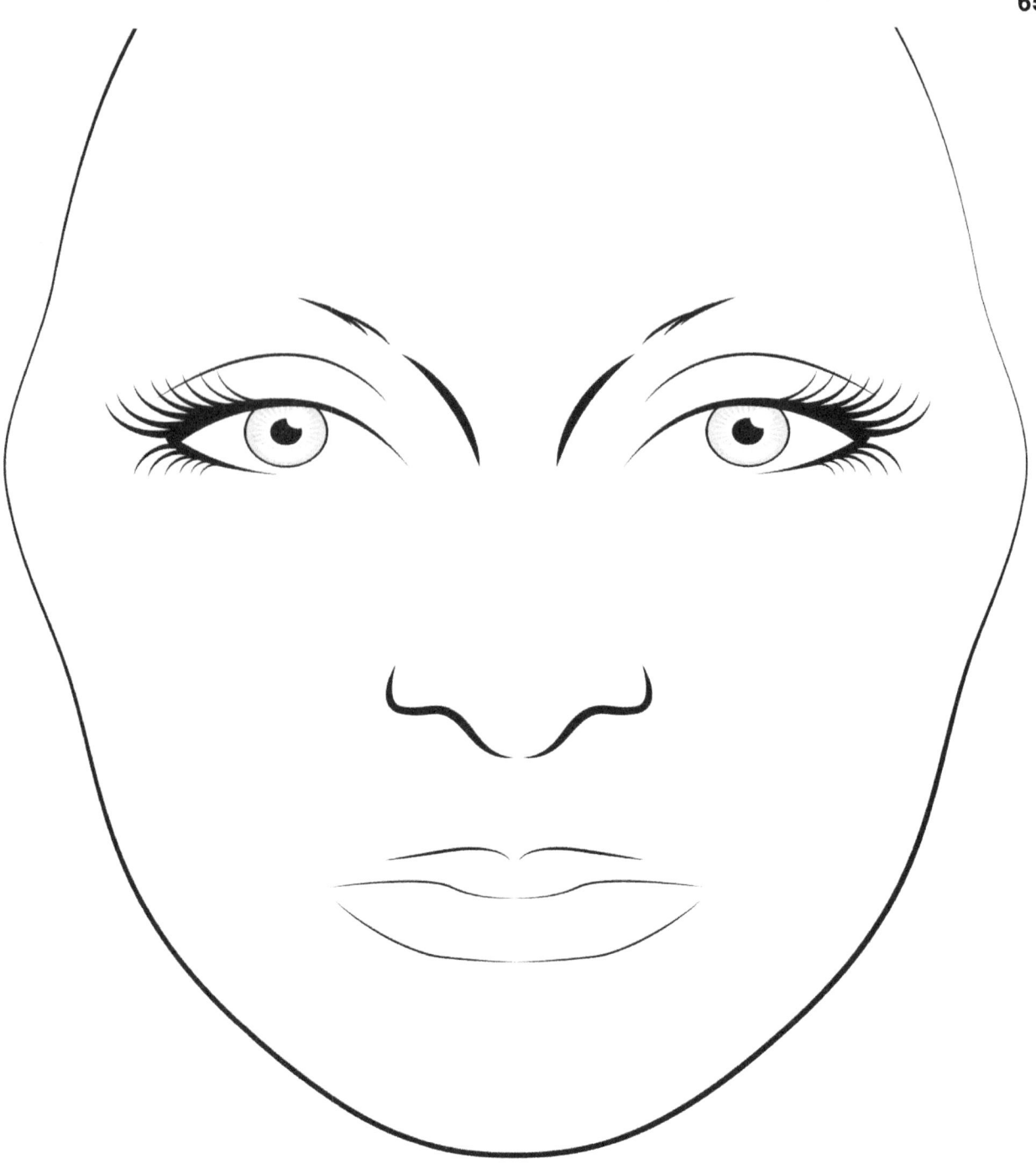

Skin	Eyes	Lips

Client Name: ....
Phone Number: ....
Email Address: ....
Makeup Look: Daytime / Evening / Wedding / Party / Other / (Circle as appropriate).

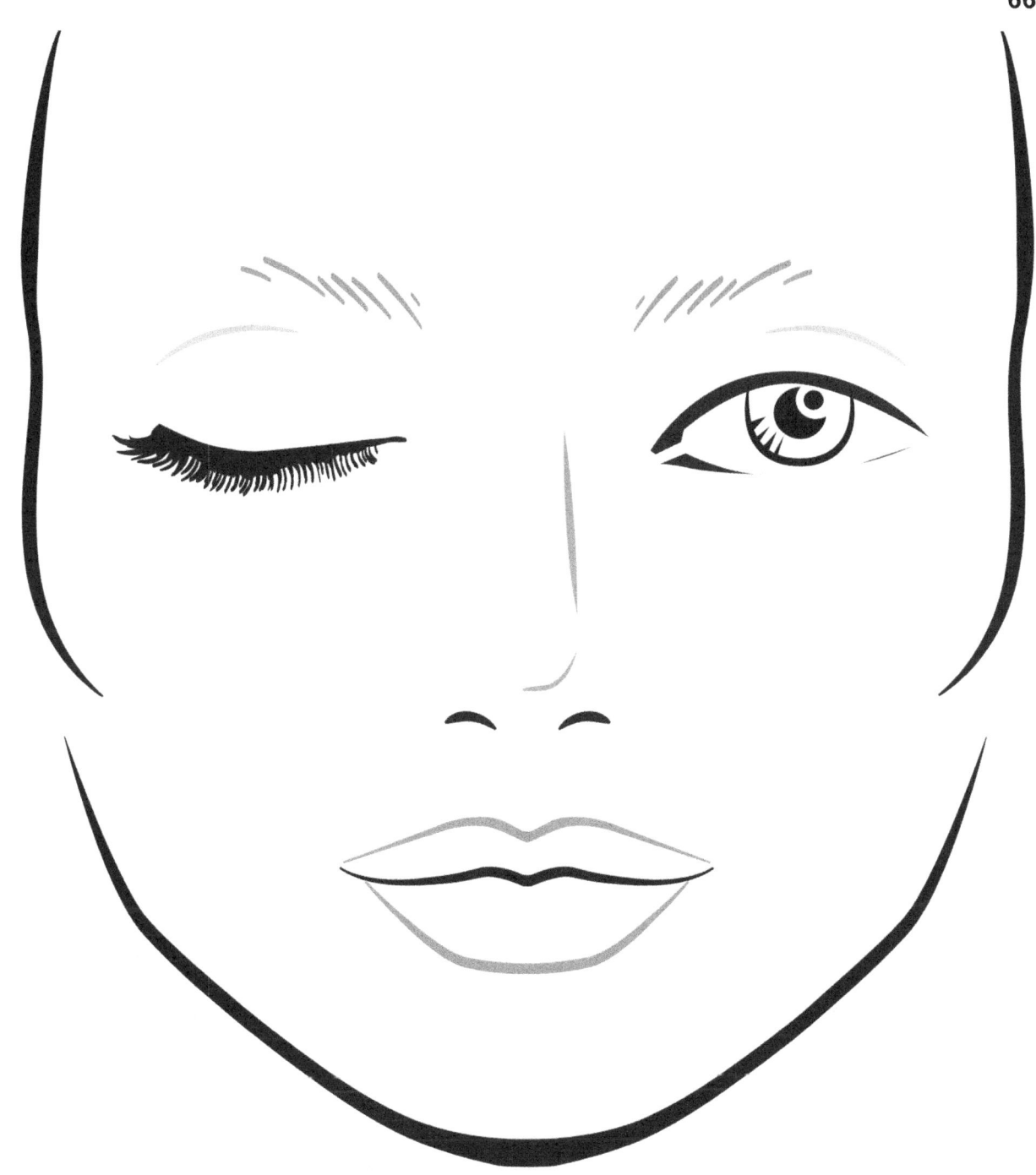

Skin	Eyes	Lips

Client Name: ....
Phone Number: ....
Email Address: ....
Makeup Look: Daytime / Evening / Wedding / Party / Other / (Circle as appropriate).

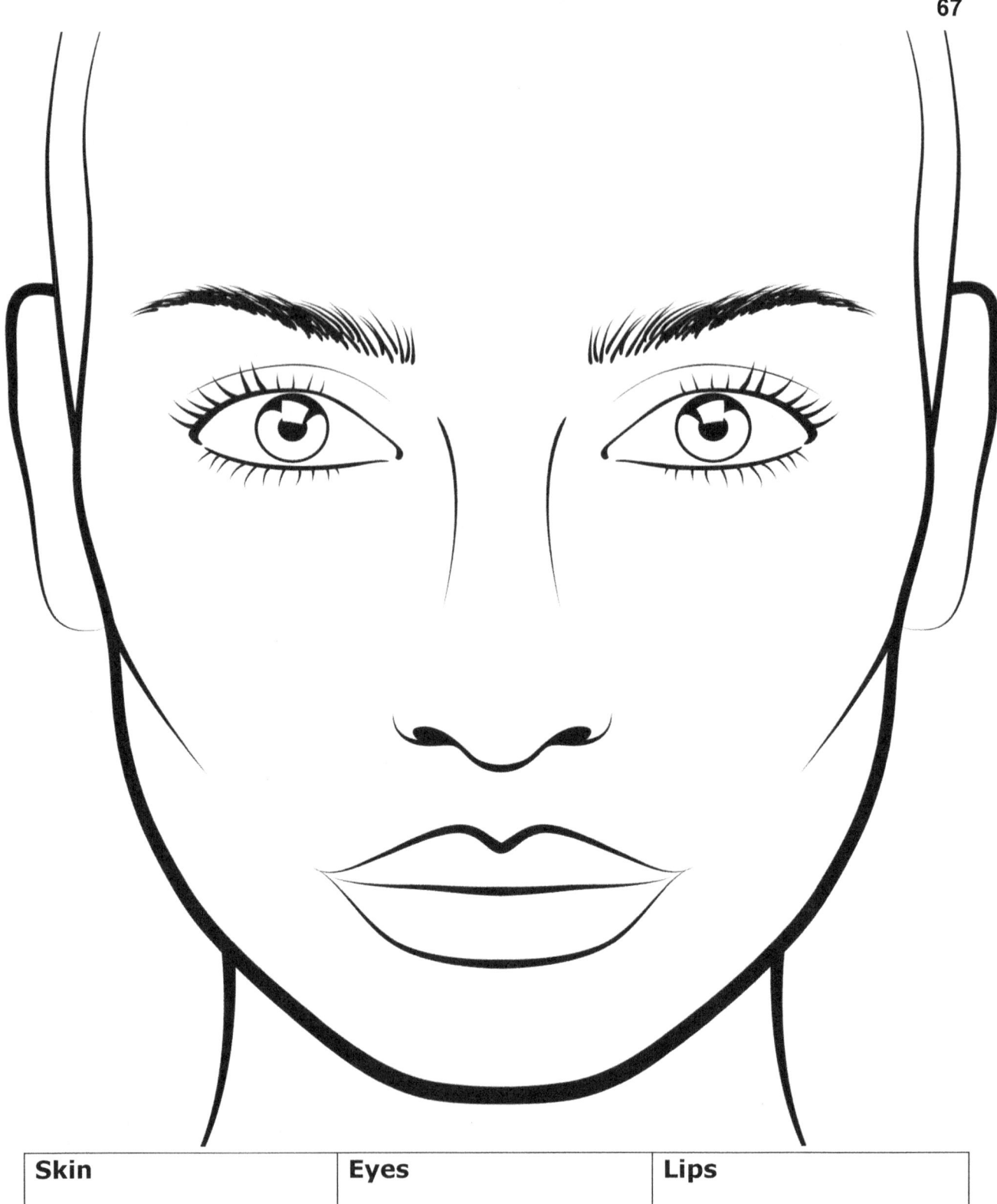

Skin	Eyes	Lips

Client Name: ....
Phone Number: ....
Email Address: ....
Makeup Look: Daytime / Evening / Wedding / Party / Other / (Circle as appropriate).

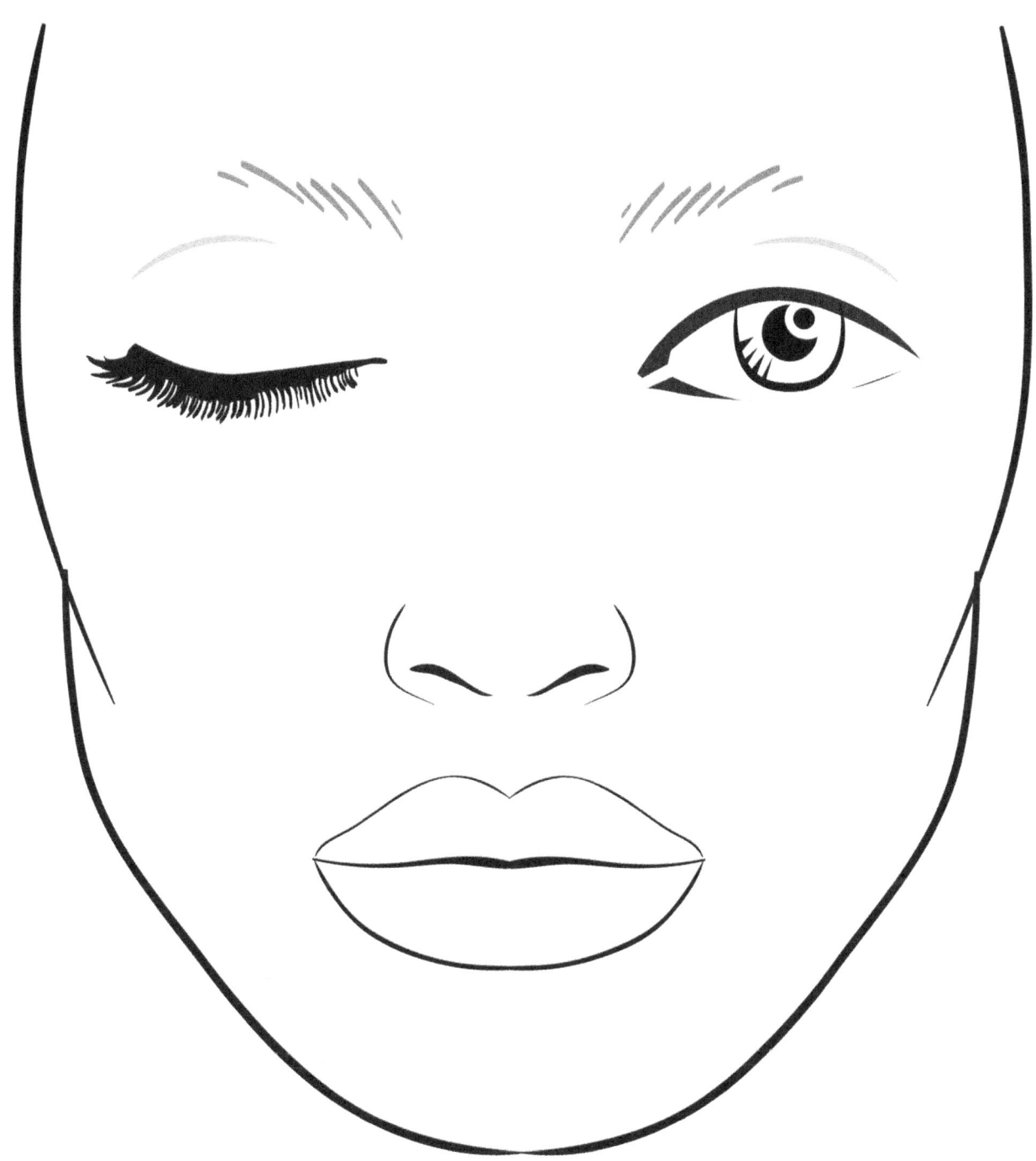

Skin	Eyes	Lips

Client Name: ....

Phone Number: ....

Email Address: ....

Makeup Look: Daytime / Evening / Wedding / Party / Other / (Circle as appropriate).

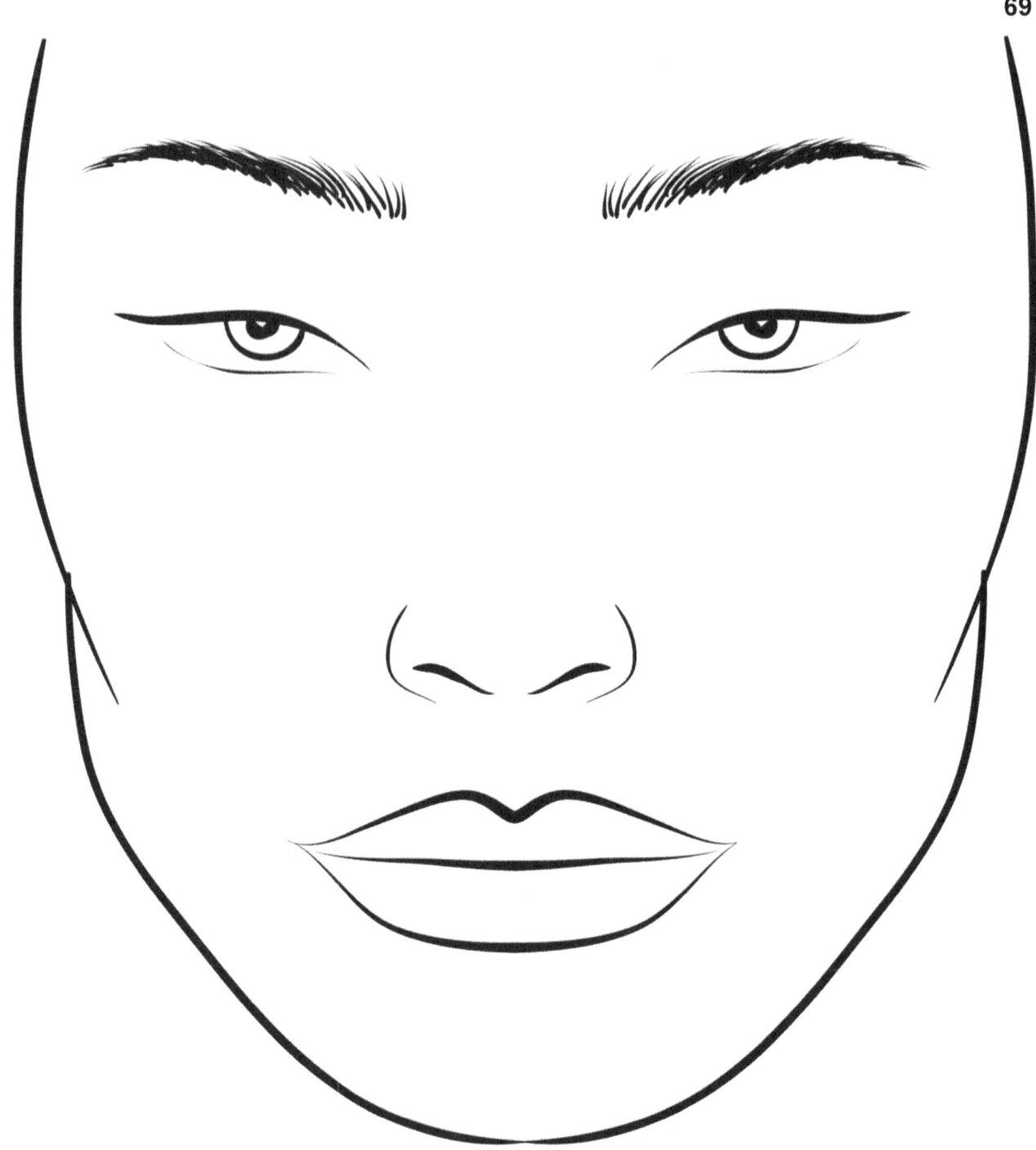

Skin	Eyes	Lips

Client Name: ....
Phone Number: ....
Email Address: ....
Makeup Look: Daytime / Evening / Wedding / Party / Other / (Circle as appropriate).

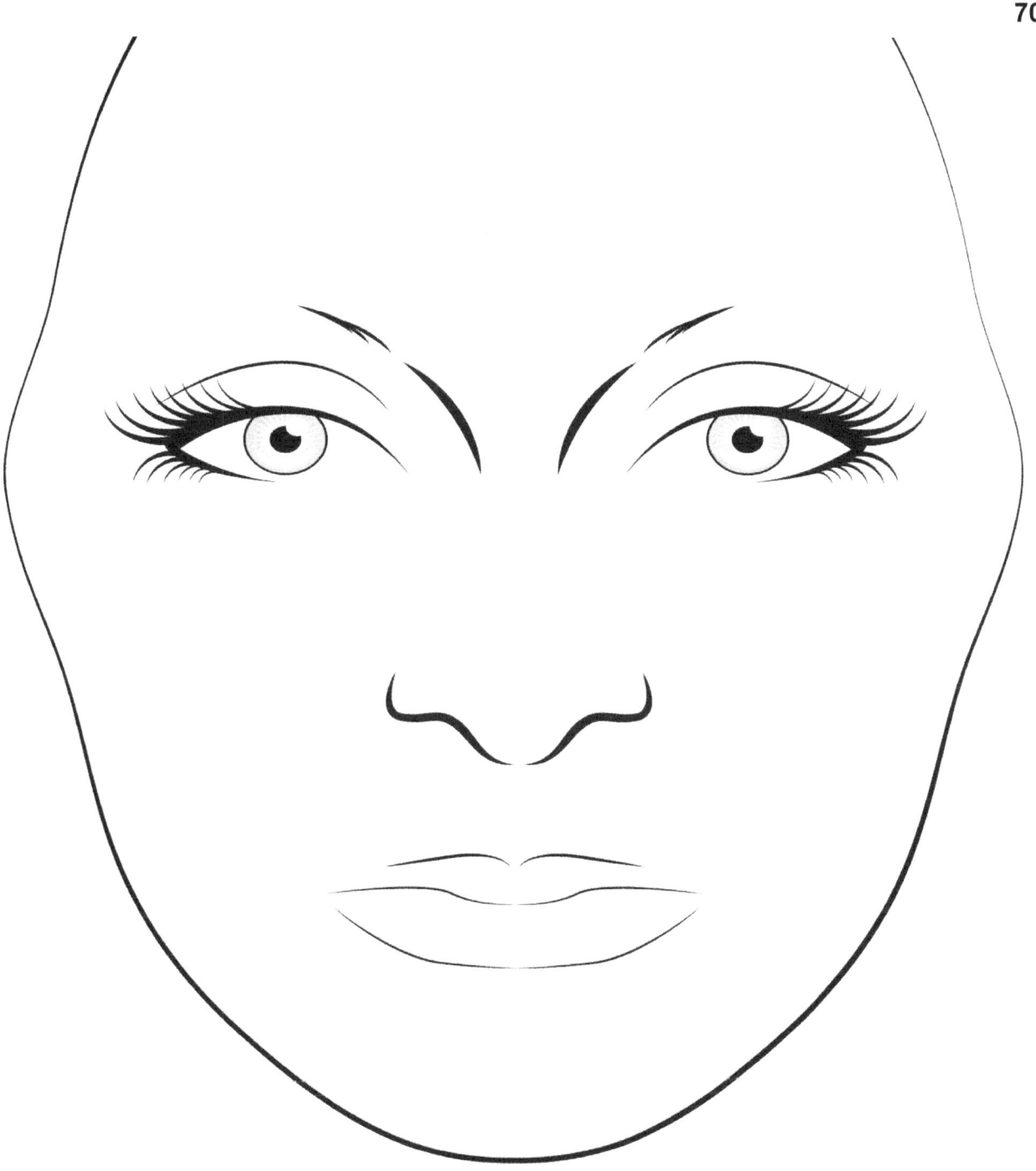

Skin	Eyes	Lips

Client Name: ....

Phone Number: ....

Email Address: ....

Makeup Look: Daytime / Evening / Wedding / Party / Other / (Circle as appropriate).

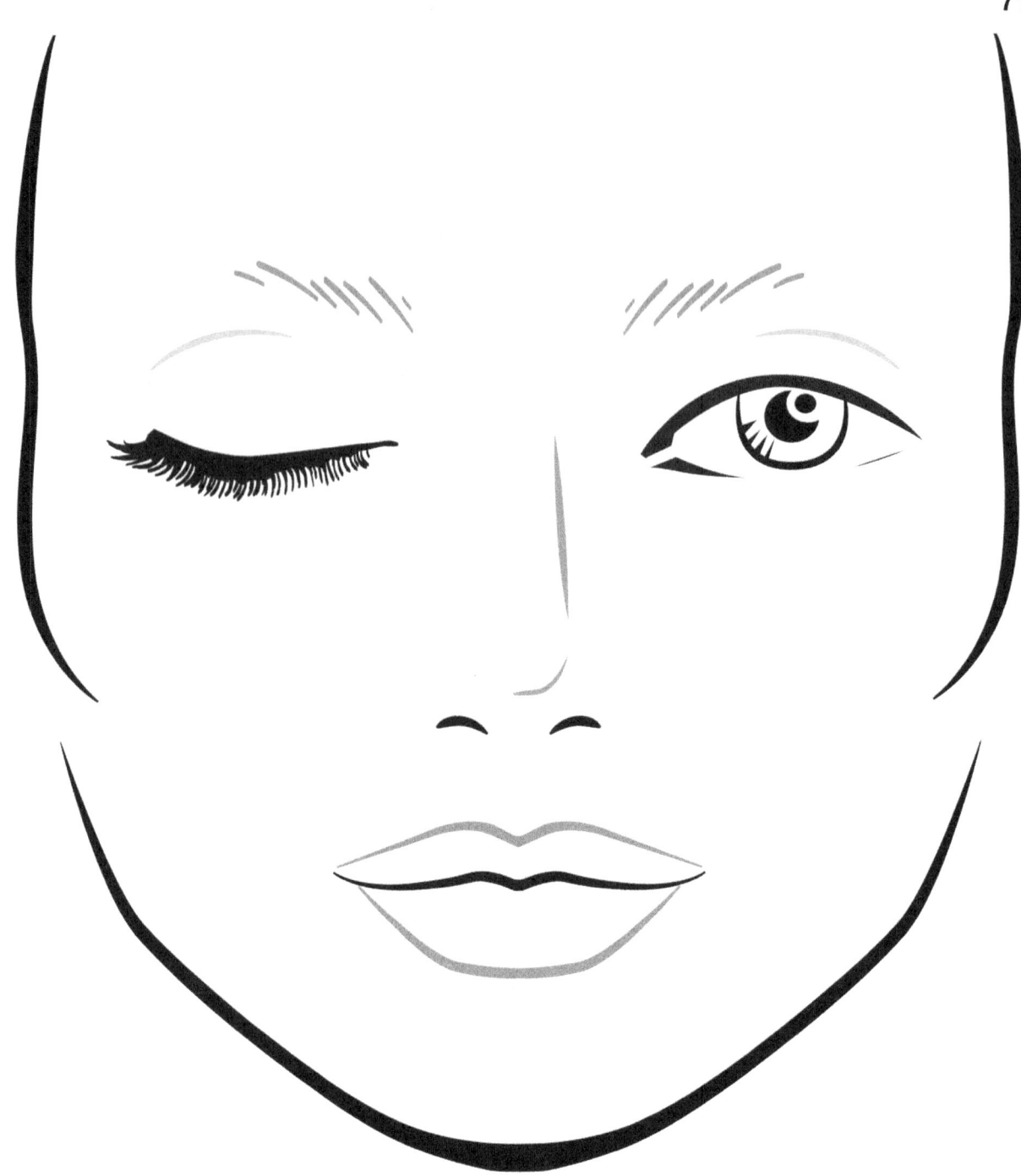

Skin	Eyes	Lips

Client Name: ....
Phone Number: ....
Email Address: ....
Makeup Look: Daytime / Evening / Wedding / Party / Other / (Circle as appropriate).

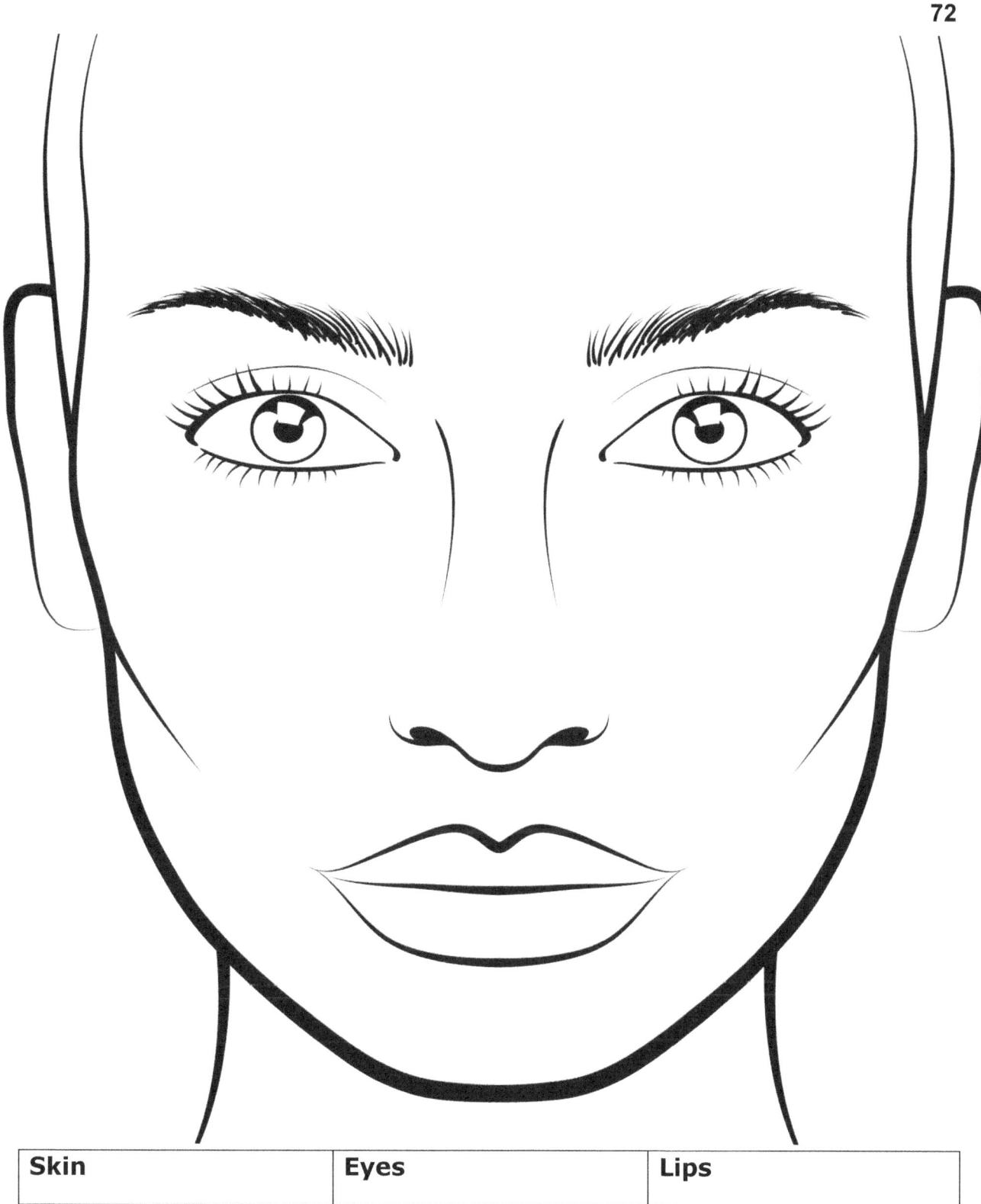

Skin	Eyes	Lips

Client Name: ....
Phone Number: ....
Email Address: ....
Makeup Look: Daytime / Evening / Wedding / Party / Other / (Circle as appropriate).

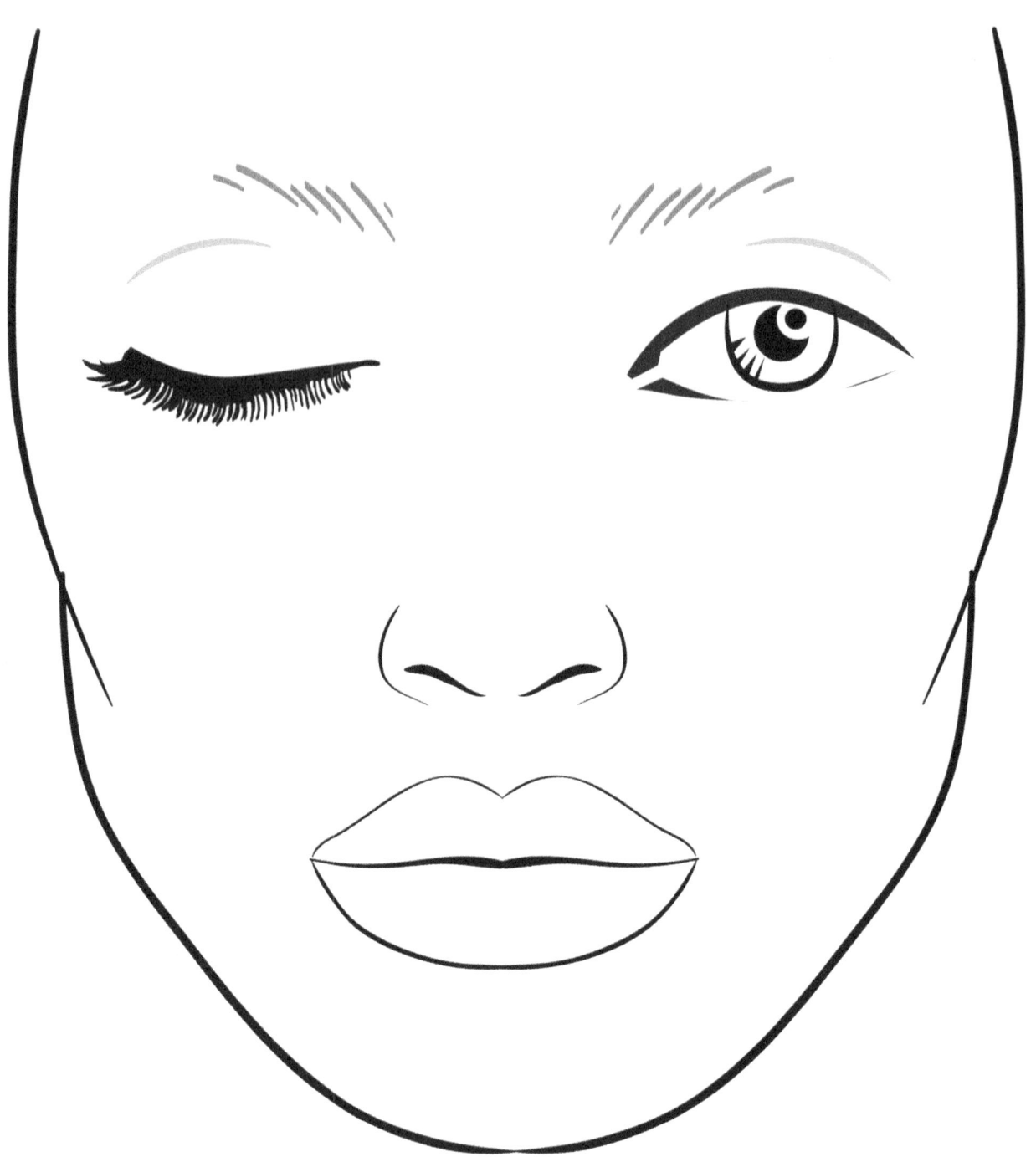

Skin	Eyes	Lips

Client Name: ....
Phone Number: ....
Email Address: ....
Makeup Look: Daytime / Evening / Wedding / Party / Other / (Circle as appropriate).

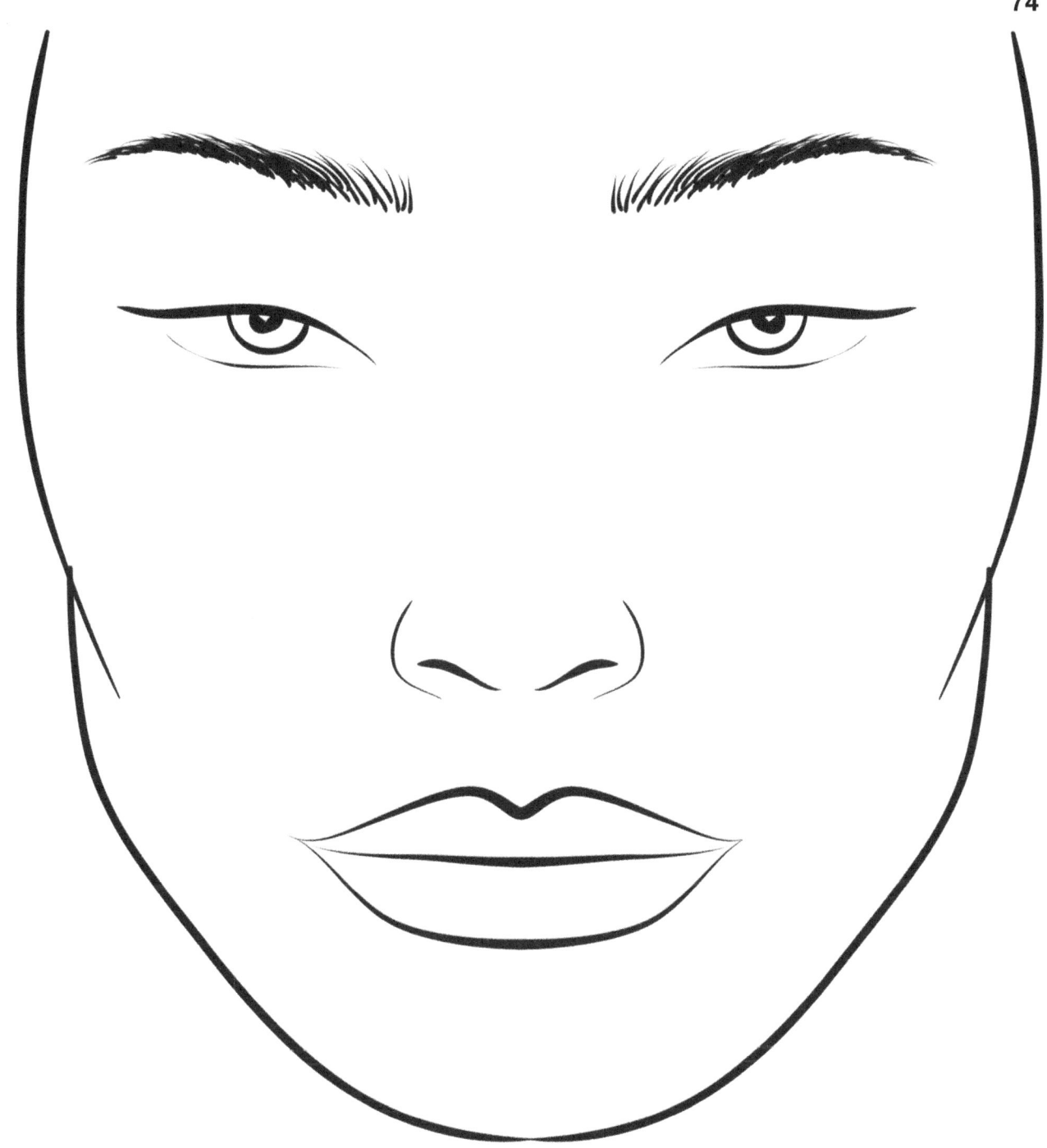

Skin	Eyes	Lips

Client Name: ....
Phone Number: ....
Email Address: ....
Makeup Look: Daytime / Evening / Wedding / Party / Other / (Circle as appropriate).

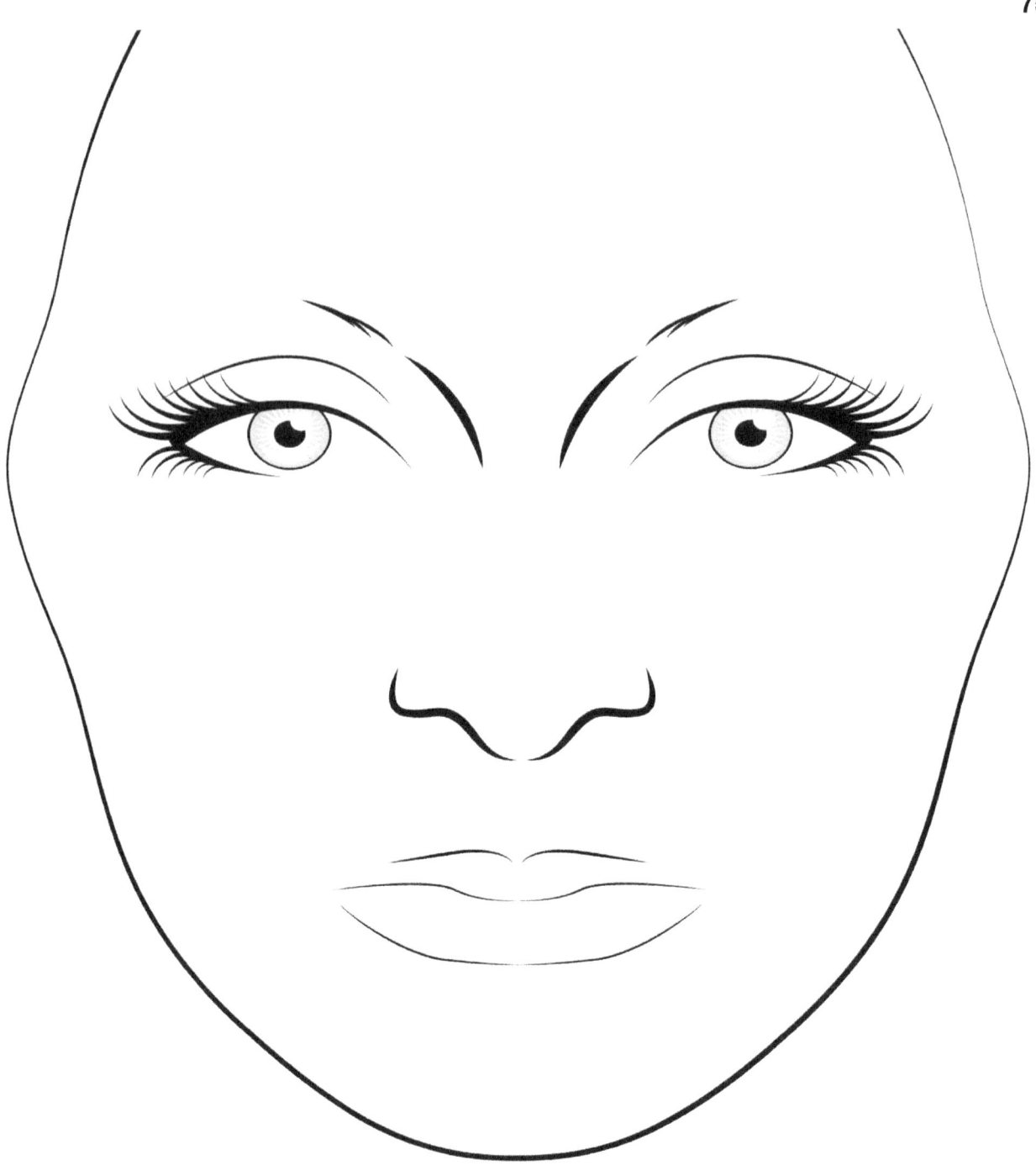

Skin	Eyes	Lips

Client Name: ....
Phone Number: ....
Email Address: ....
Makeup Look: Daytime / Evening / Wedding / Party / Other / (Circle as appropriate).

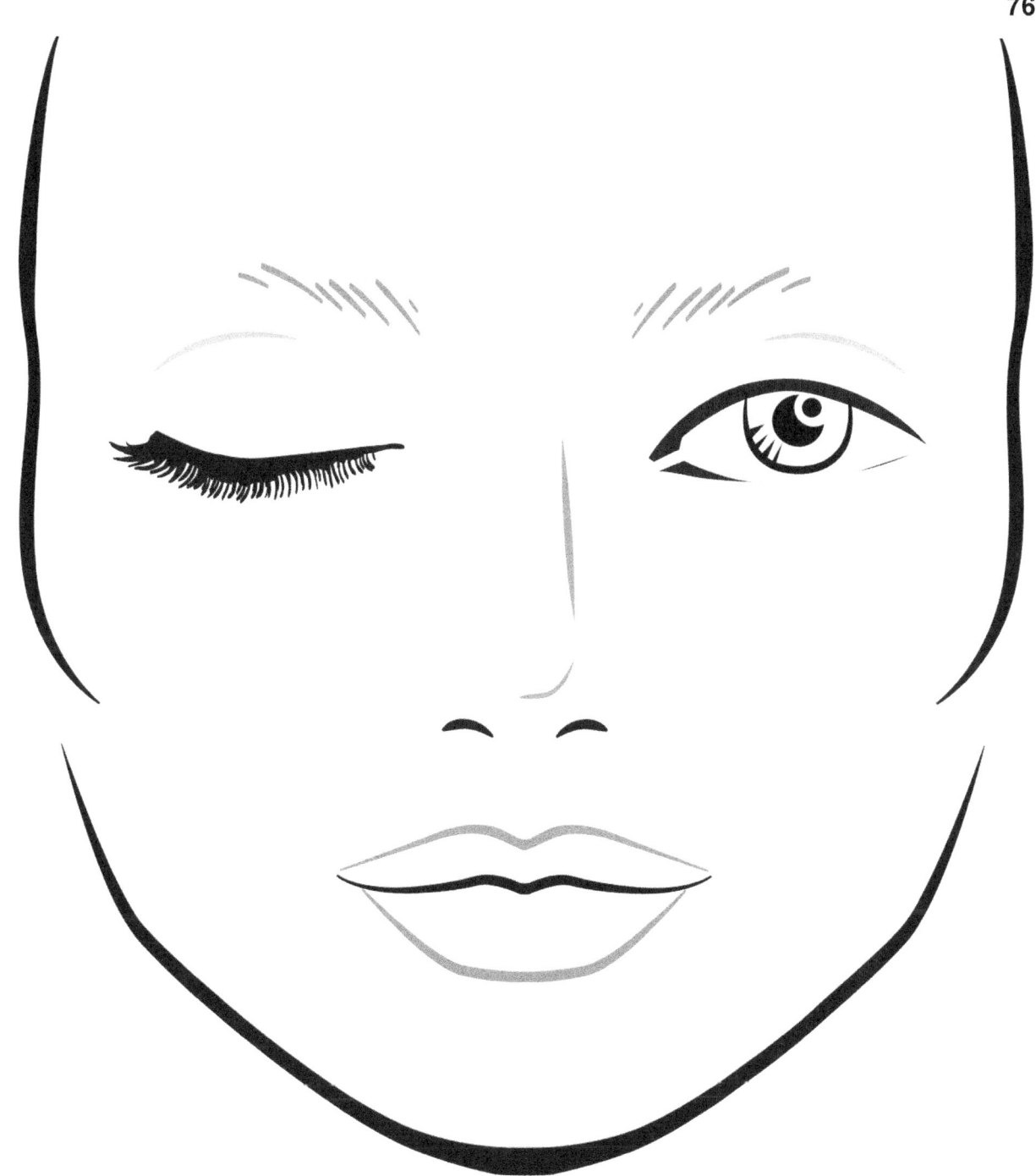

Skin	Eyes	Lips

Client Name: ....
Phone Number: ....
Email Address: ....
Makeup Look: Daytime / Evening / Wedding / Party / Other / (Circle as appropriate).

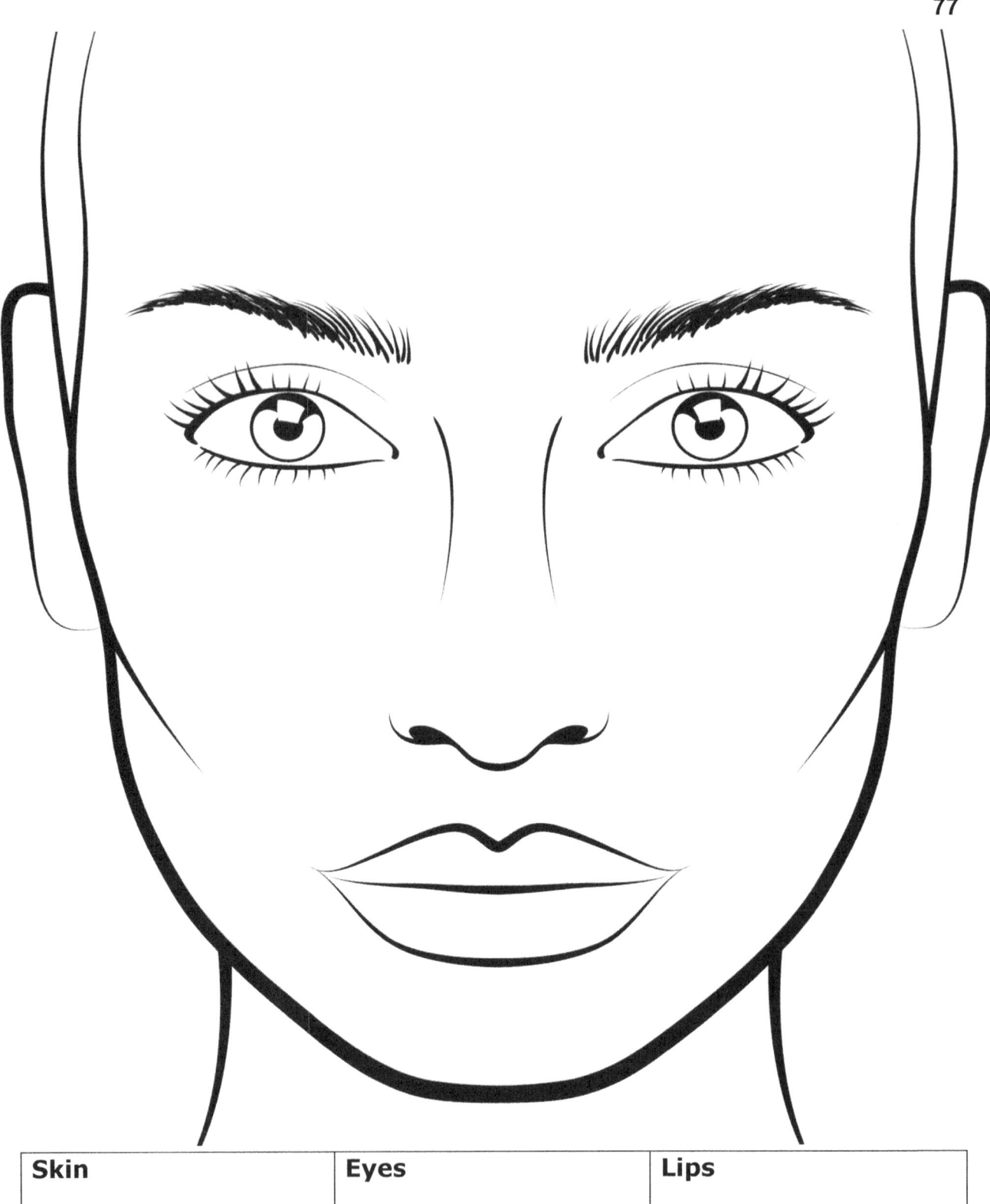

Skin	Eyes	Lips

Client Name: ....
Phone Number: ....
Email Address: ....
Makeup Look: Daytime / Evening / Wedding / Party / Other / (Circle as appropriate).

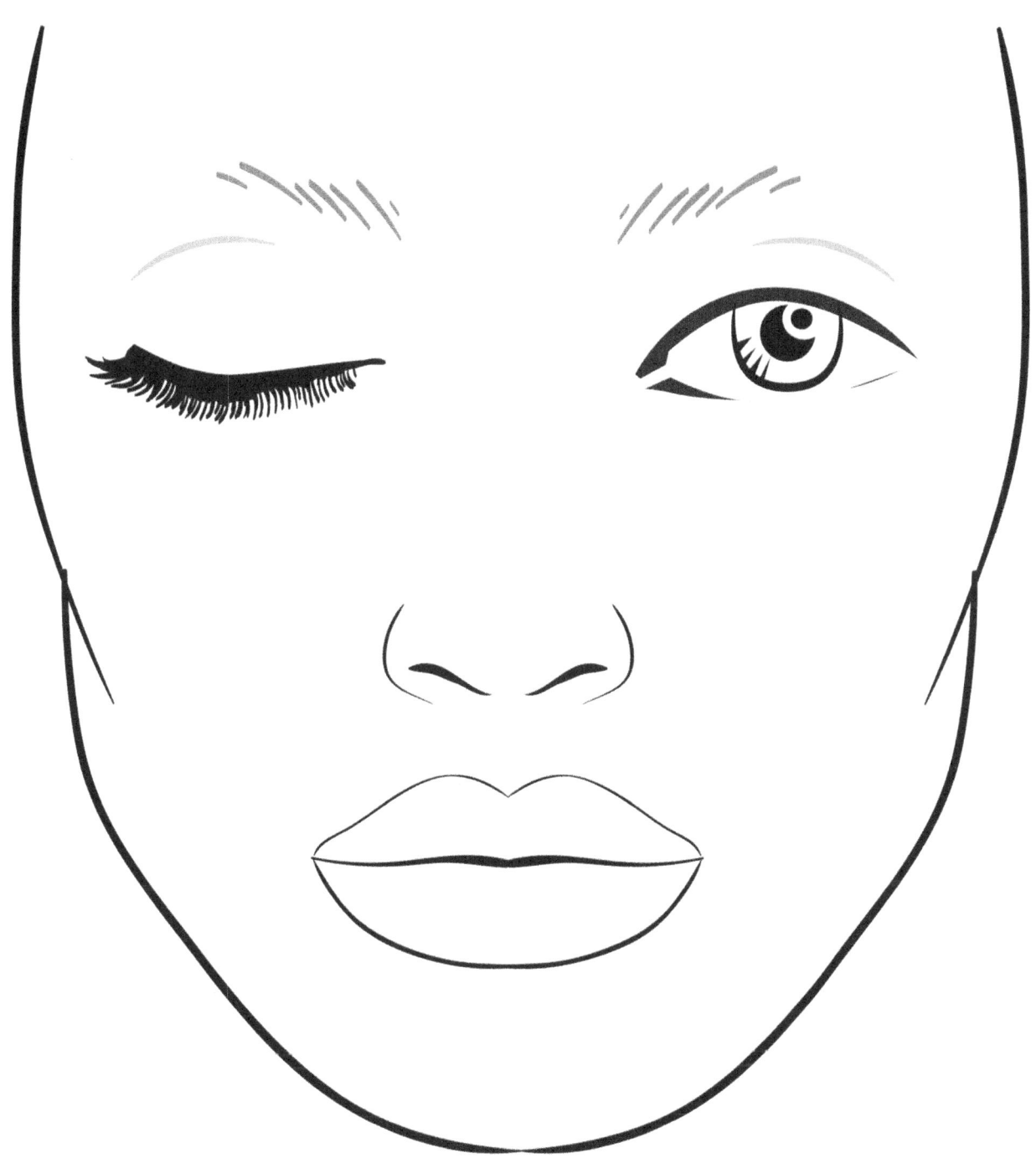

Skin	Eyes	Lips

Client Name: ....
Phone Number: ....
Email Address: ....
Makeup Look: Daytime / Evening / Wedding / Party / Other / (Circle as appropriate).

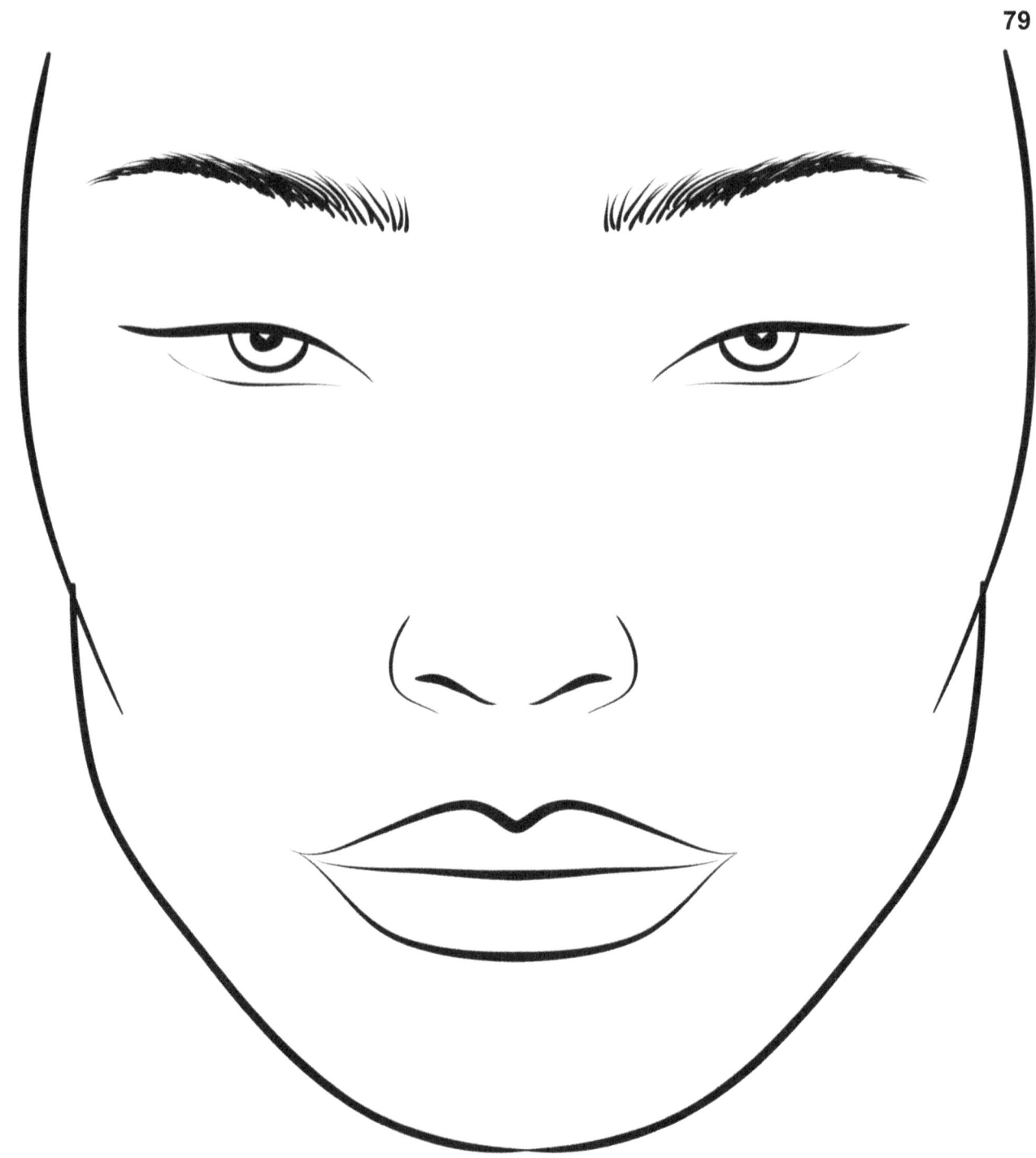

Skin	Eyes	Lips

Client Name: ....

Phone Number: ....

Email Address: ....

Makeup Look: Daytime / Evening / Wedding / Party / Other / (Circle as appropriate).

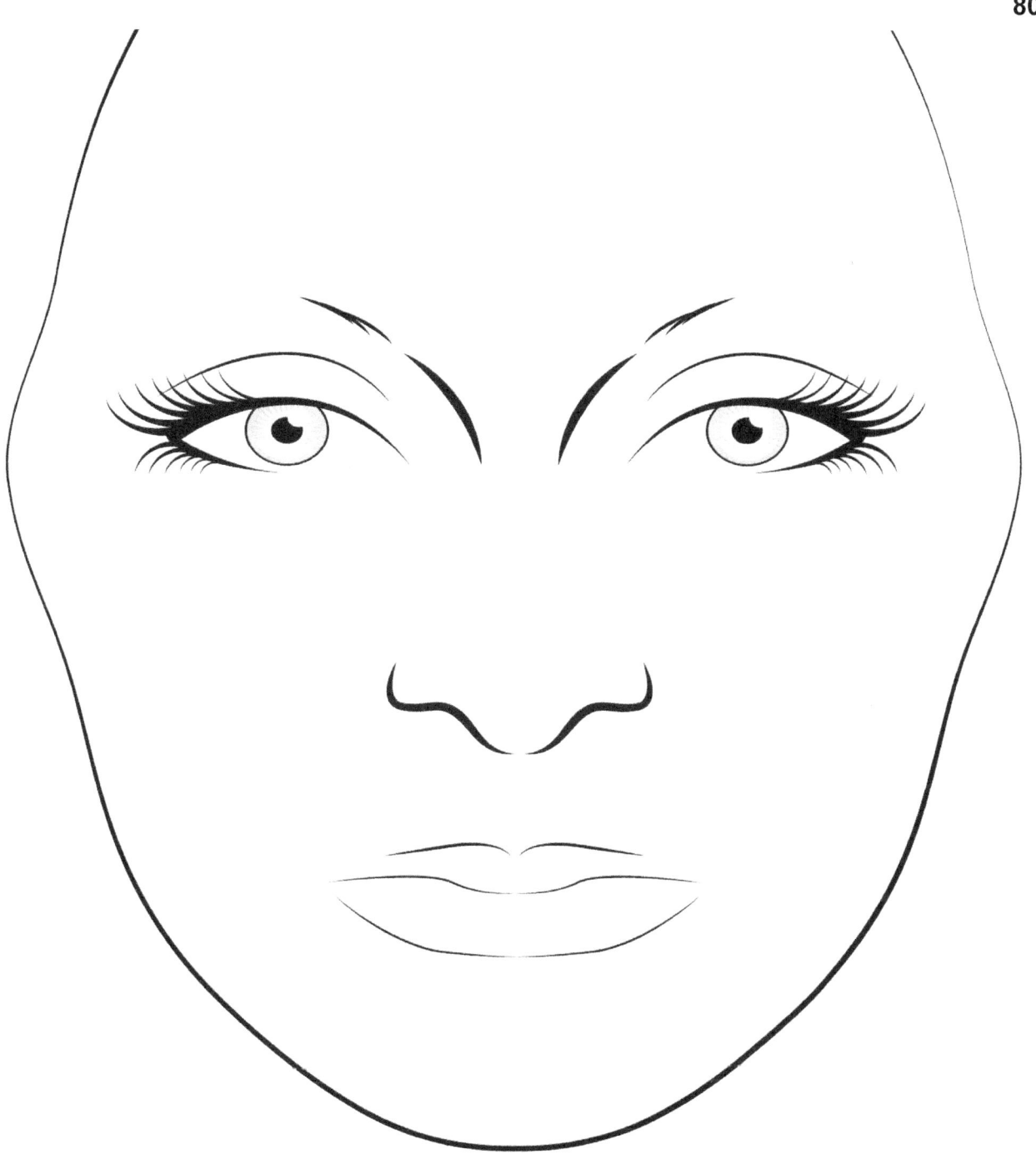

Skin	Eyes	Lips

Client Name: ....
Phone Number: ....
Email Address: ....
Makeup Look: Daytime / Evening / Wedding / Party / Other / (Circle as appropriate).

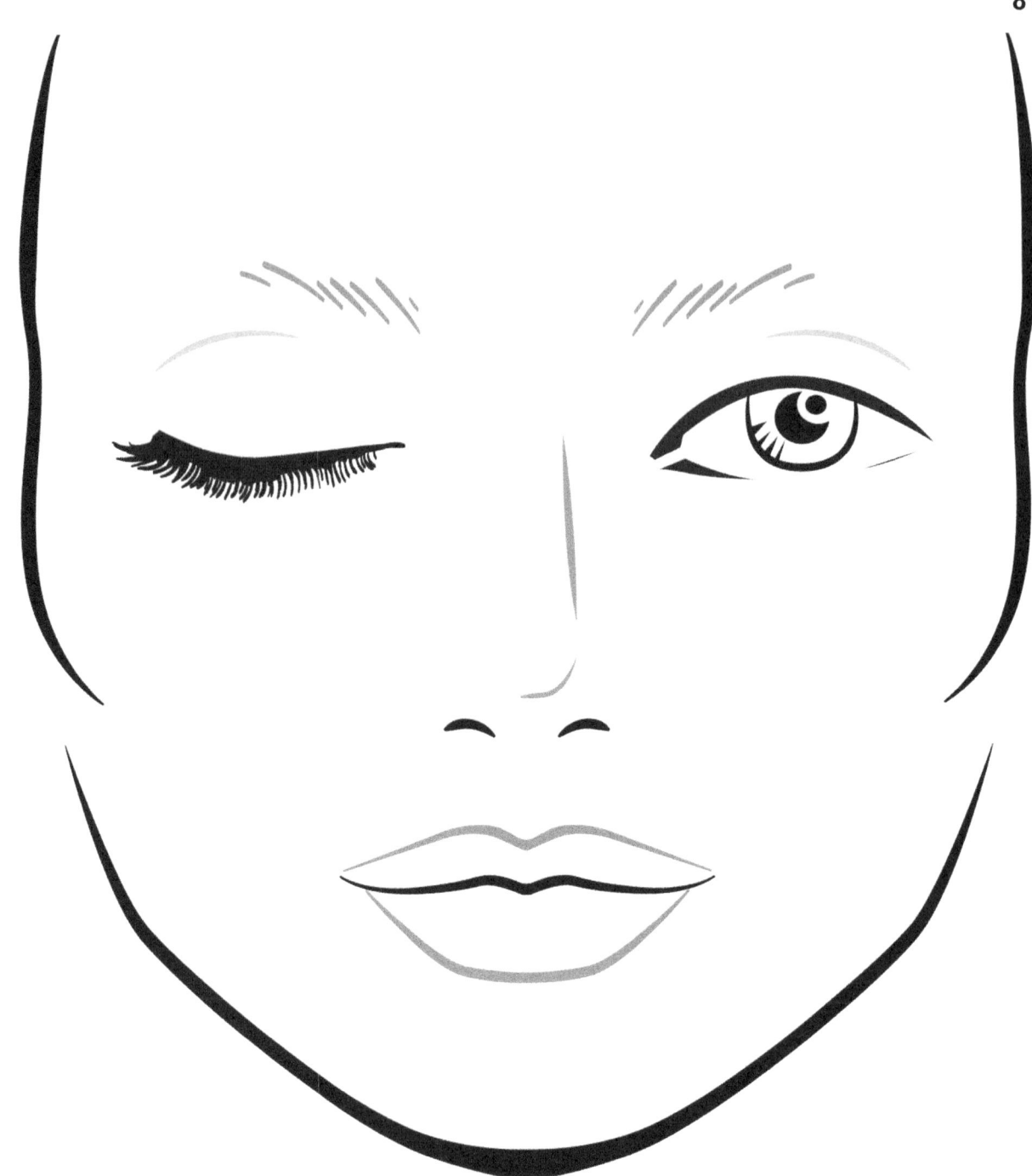

Skin	Eyes	Lips

Client Name: ....
Phone Number: ....
Email Address: ....
Makeup Look: Daytime / Evening / Wedding / Party / Other / (Circle as appropriate).

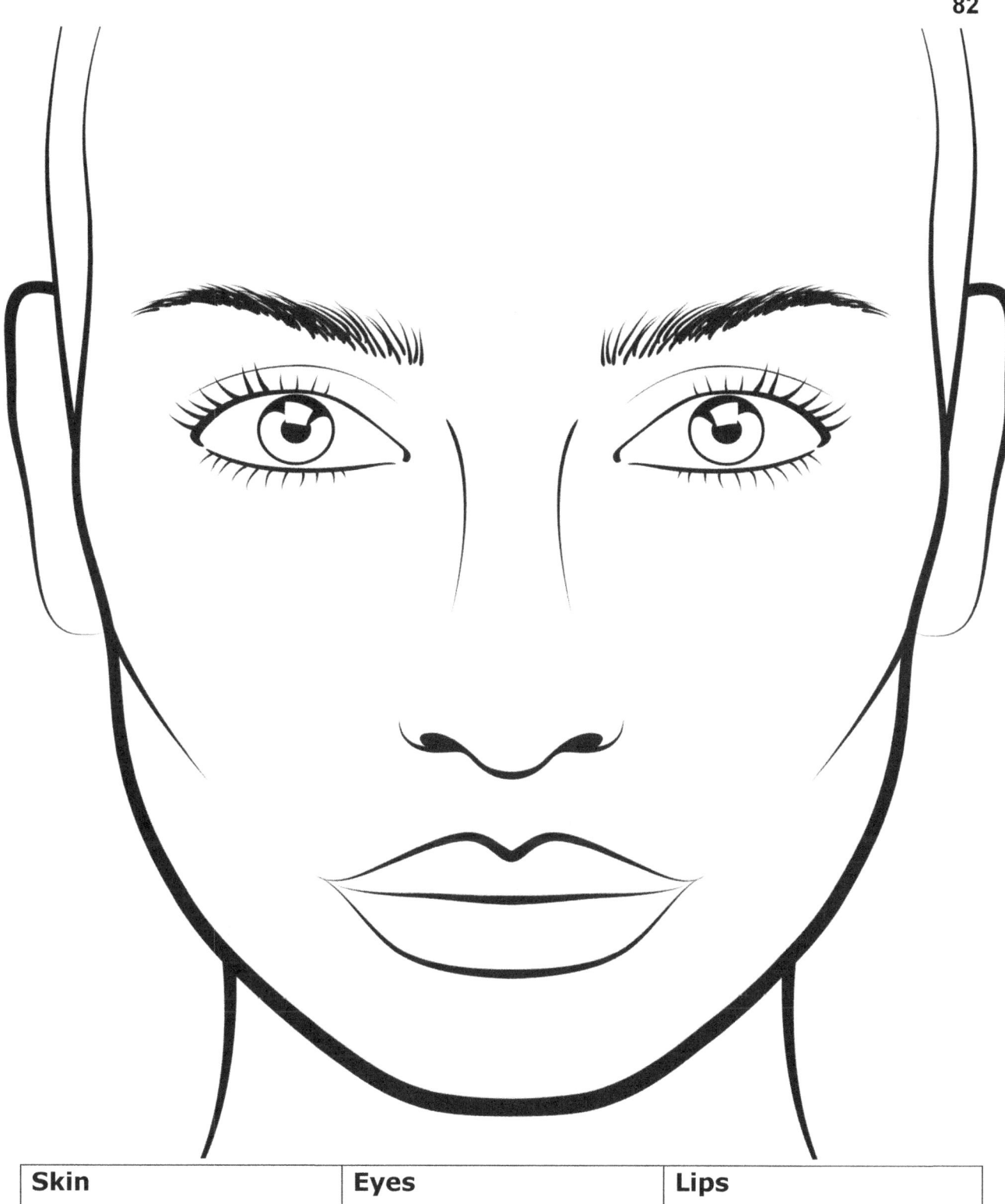

Skin	Eyes	Lips

Client Name: ....
Phone Number: ....
Email Address: ....
Makeup Look: Daytime / Evening / Wedding / Party / Other / (Circle as appropriate).

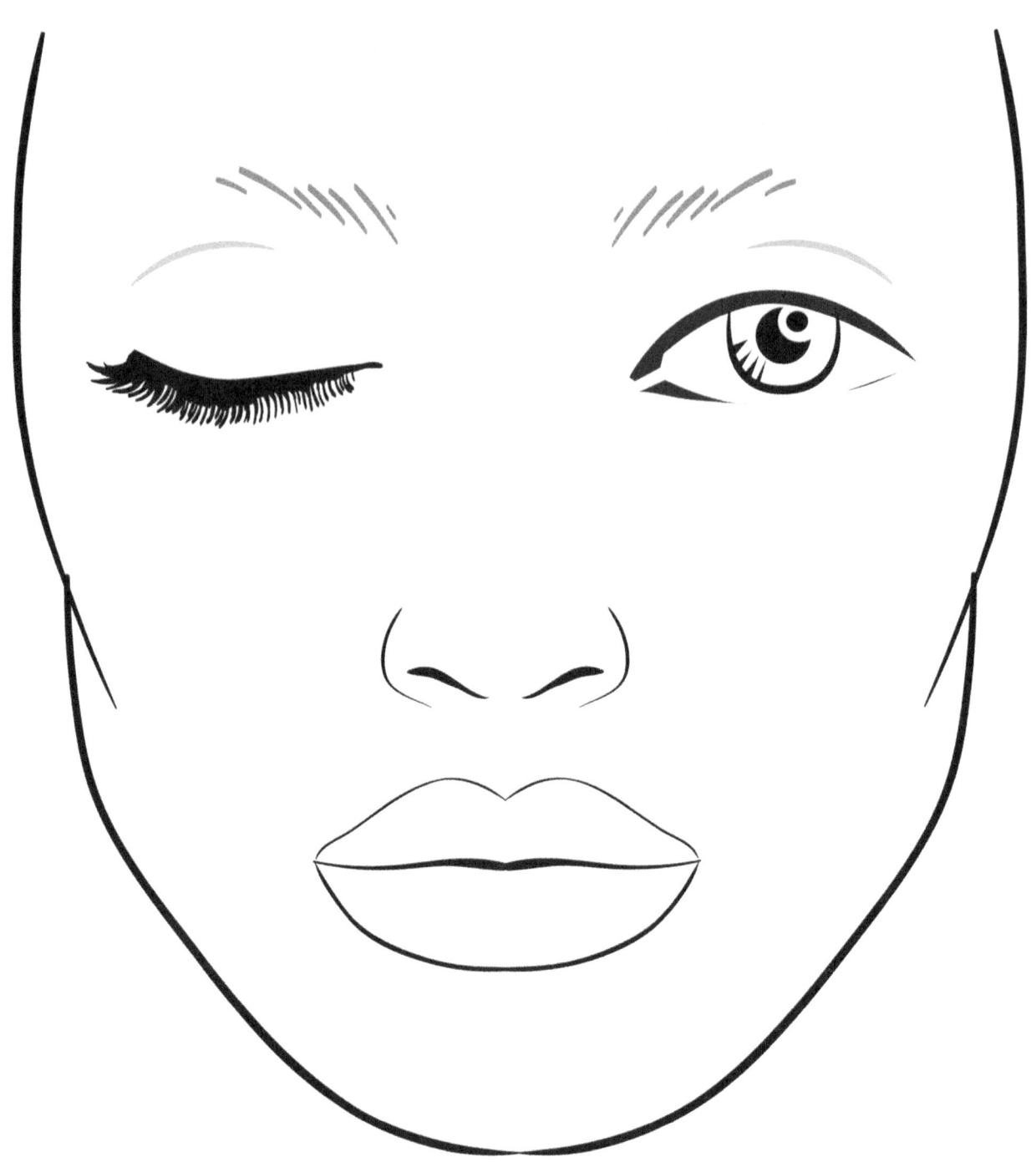

Skin	Eyes	Lips

Client Name: ....

Phone Number: ....

Email Address: ....

Makeup Look: Daytime / Evening / Wedding / Party / Other / (Circle as appropriate).

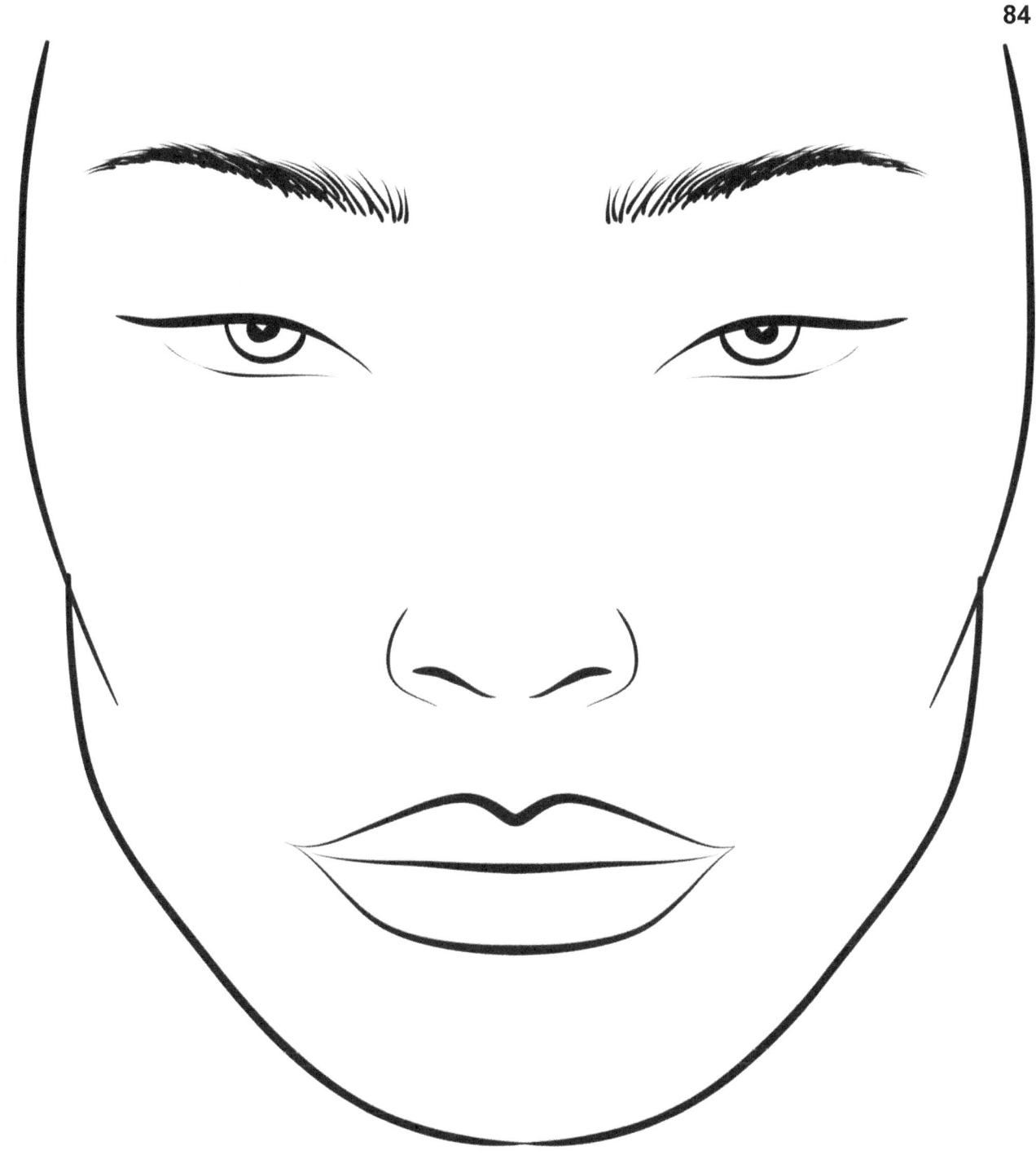

Skin	Eyes	Lips

Client Name: ....
Phone Number: ....
Email Address: ....
Makeup Look: Daytime / Evening / Wedding / Party / Other / (Circle as appropriate).

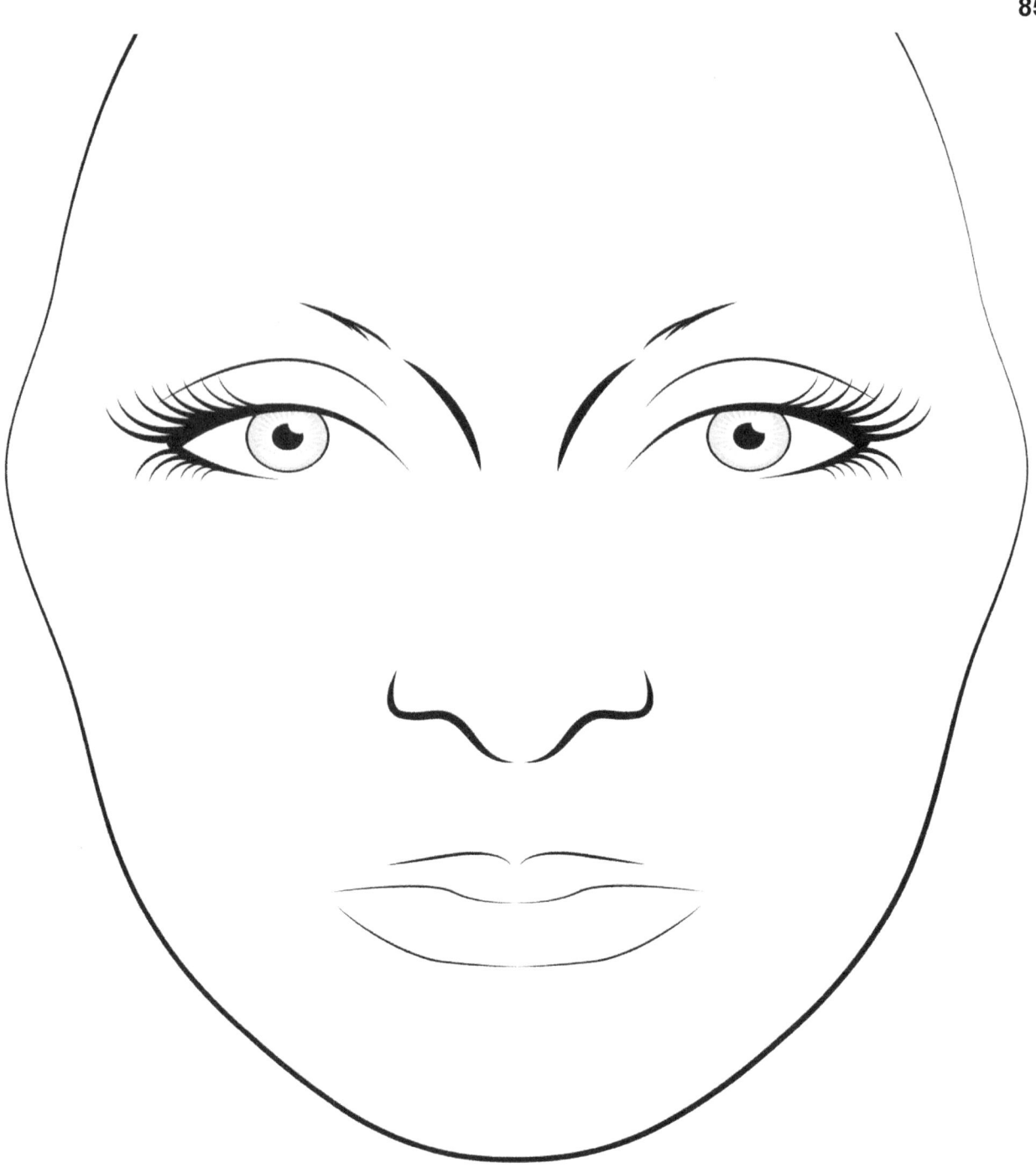

Skin	Eyes	Lips

Client Name: ....
Phone Number: ....
Email Address: ....
Makeup Look: Daytime / Evening / Wedding / Party / Other / (Circle as appropriate).

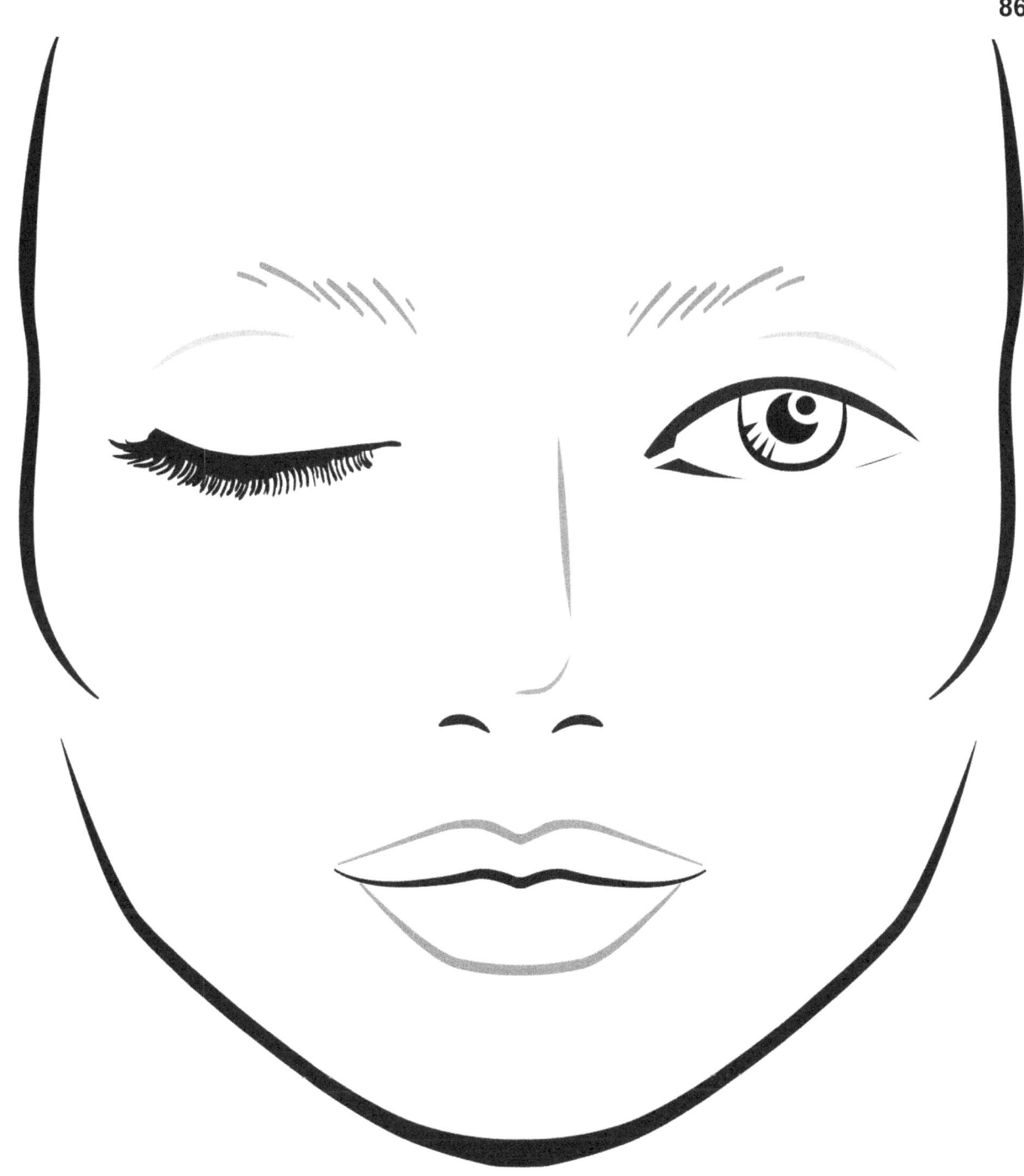

Skin	Eyes	Lips

Client Name: ....
Phone Number: ....
Email Address: ....
Makeup Look: Daytime / Evening / Wedding / Party / Other / (Circle as appropriate).

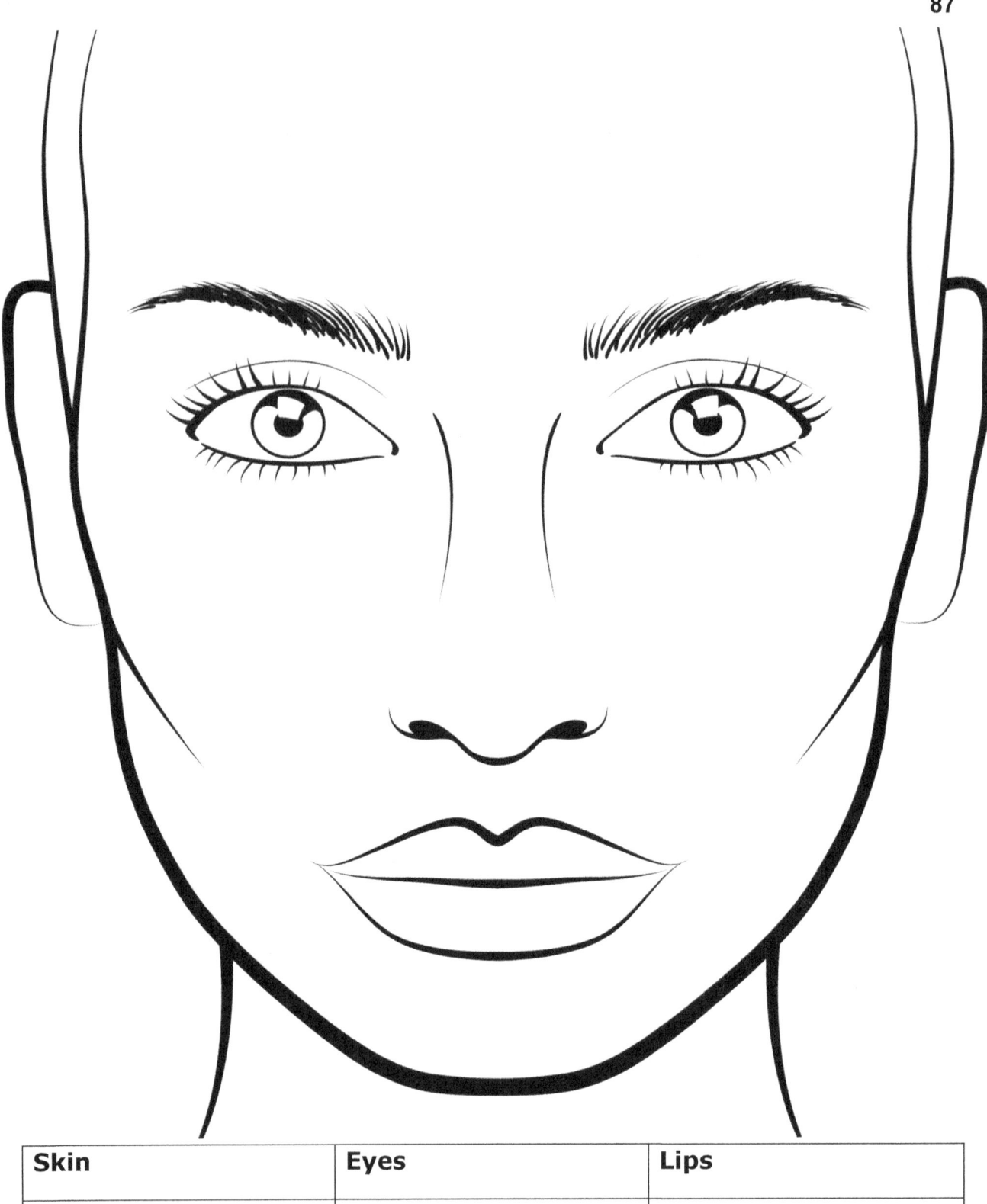

Skin	Eyes	Lips

Client Name: ....
Phone Number: ....
Email Address: ....
Makeup Look: Daytime / Evening / Wedding / Party / Other / (Circle as appropriate).

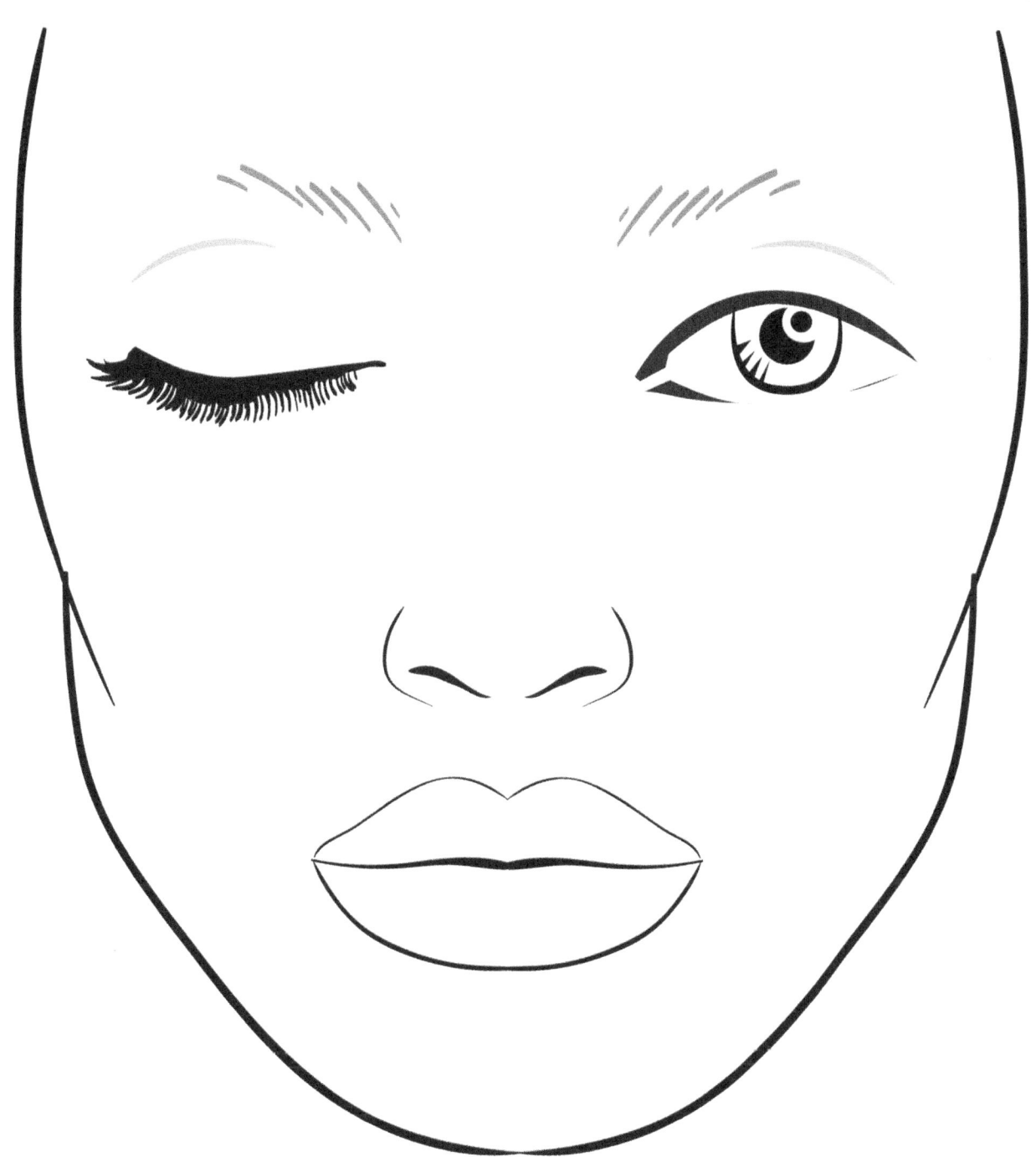

Skin	Eyes	Lips

Client Name: ....
Phone Number: ....
Email Address: ....
Makeup Look: Daytime / Evening / Wedding / Party / Other / (Circle as appropriate).

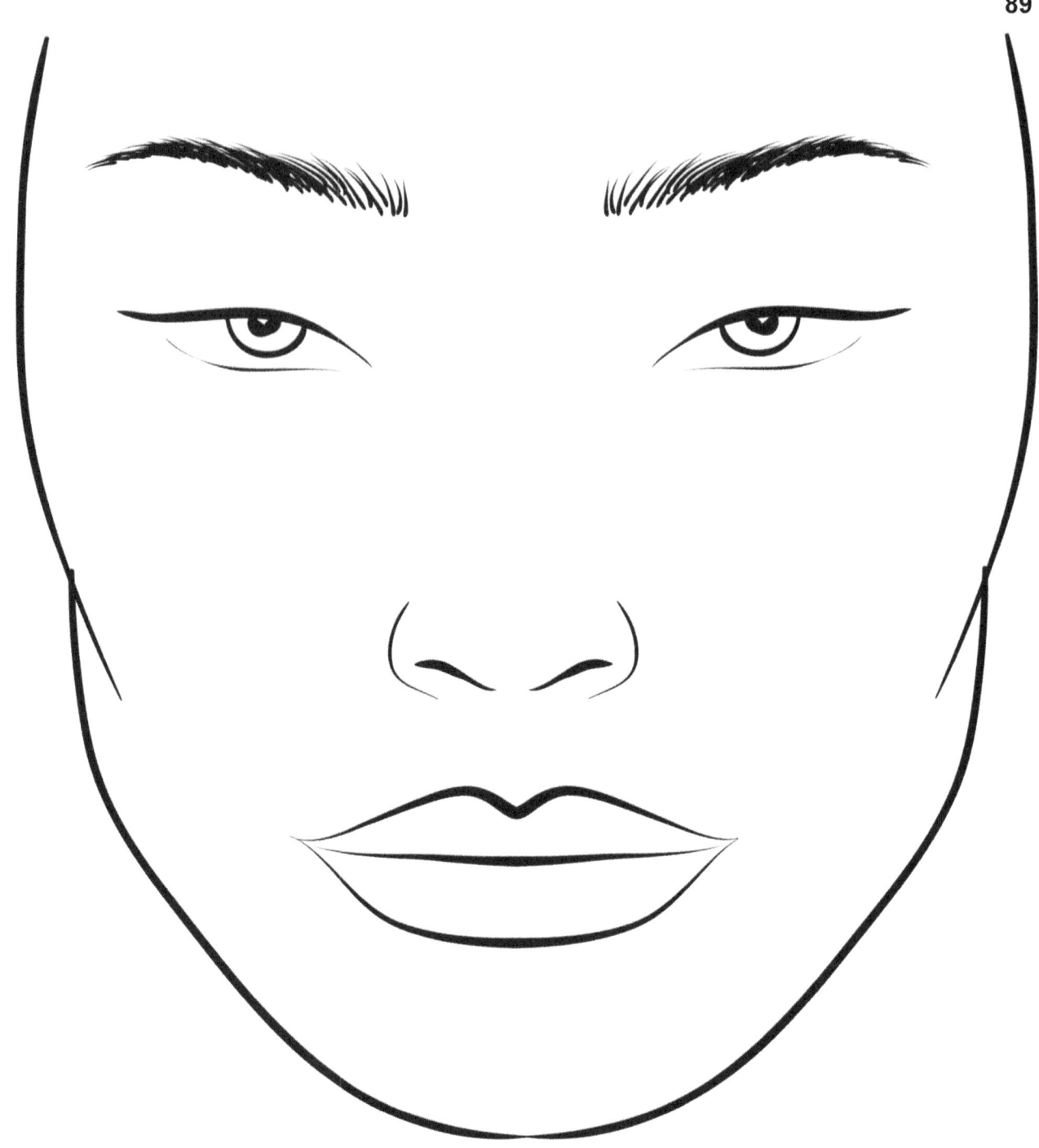

Skin	Eyes	Lips

Client Name: ....
Phone Number: ....
Email Address: ....
Makeup Look: Daytime / Evening / Wedding / Party / Other / (Circle as appropriate).

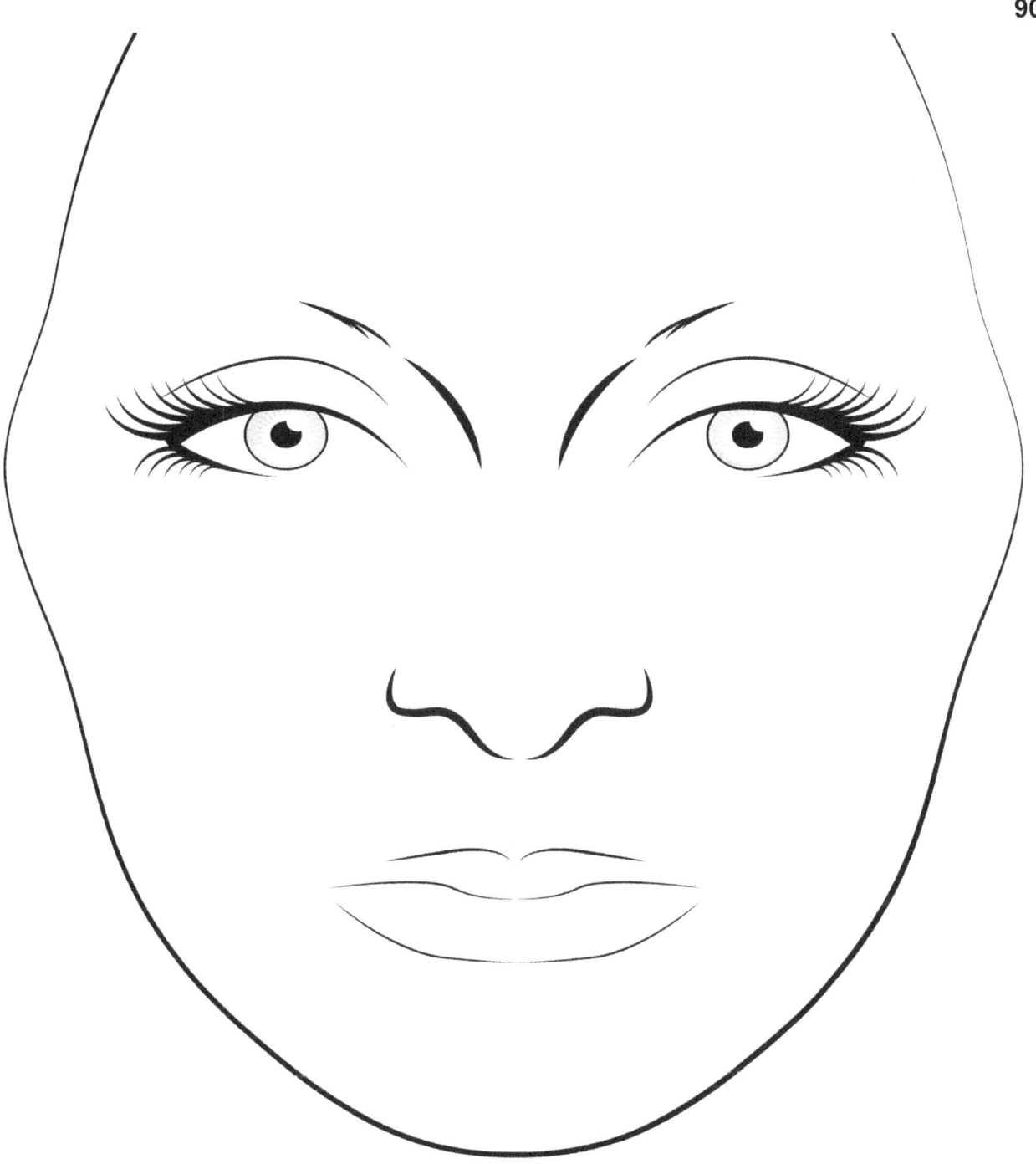

Skin	Eyes	Lips

Client Name: ....
Phone Number: ....
Email Address: ....
Makeup Look: Daytime / Evening / Wedding / Party / Other / (Circle as appropriate).

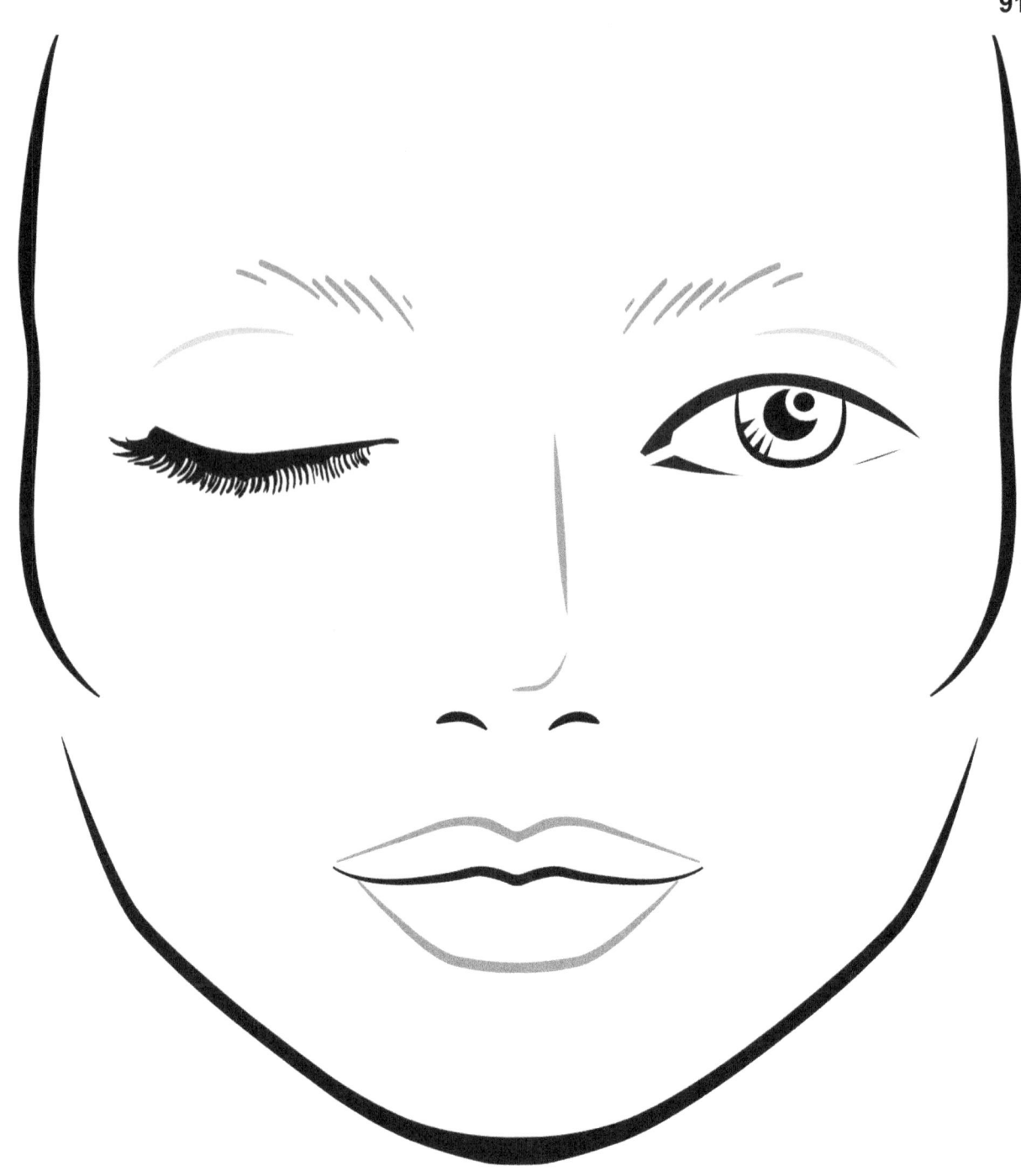

Skin	Eyes	Lips

Client Name: ....
Phone Number: ....
Email Address: ....
Makeup Look: Daytime / Evening / Wedding / Party / Other / (Circle as appropriate).

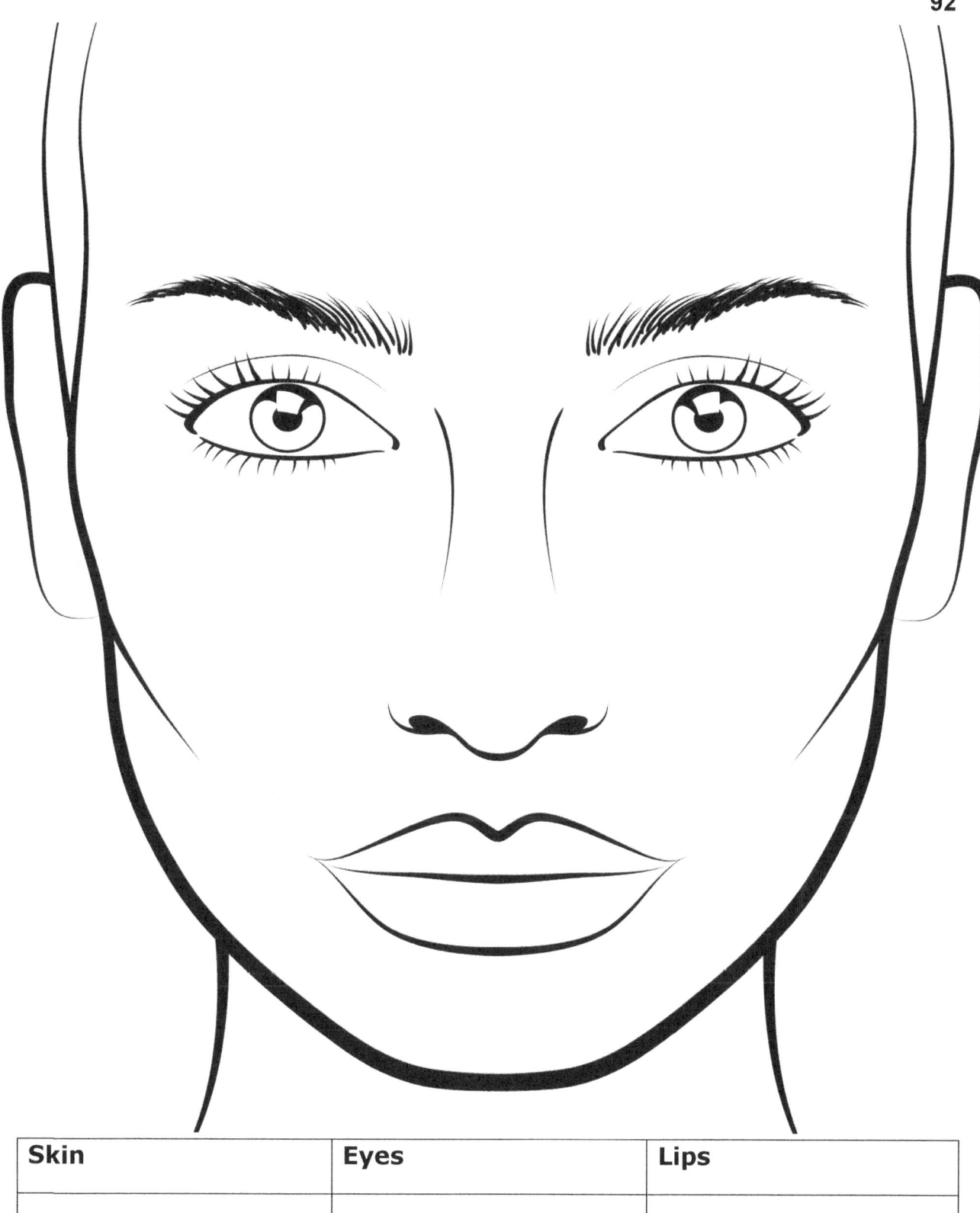

Skin	Eyes	Lips

Client Name: ....
Phone Number: ....
Email Address: ....
Makeup Look: Daytime / Evening / Wedding / Party / Other / (Circle as appropriate).

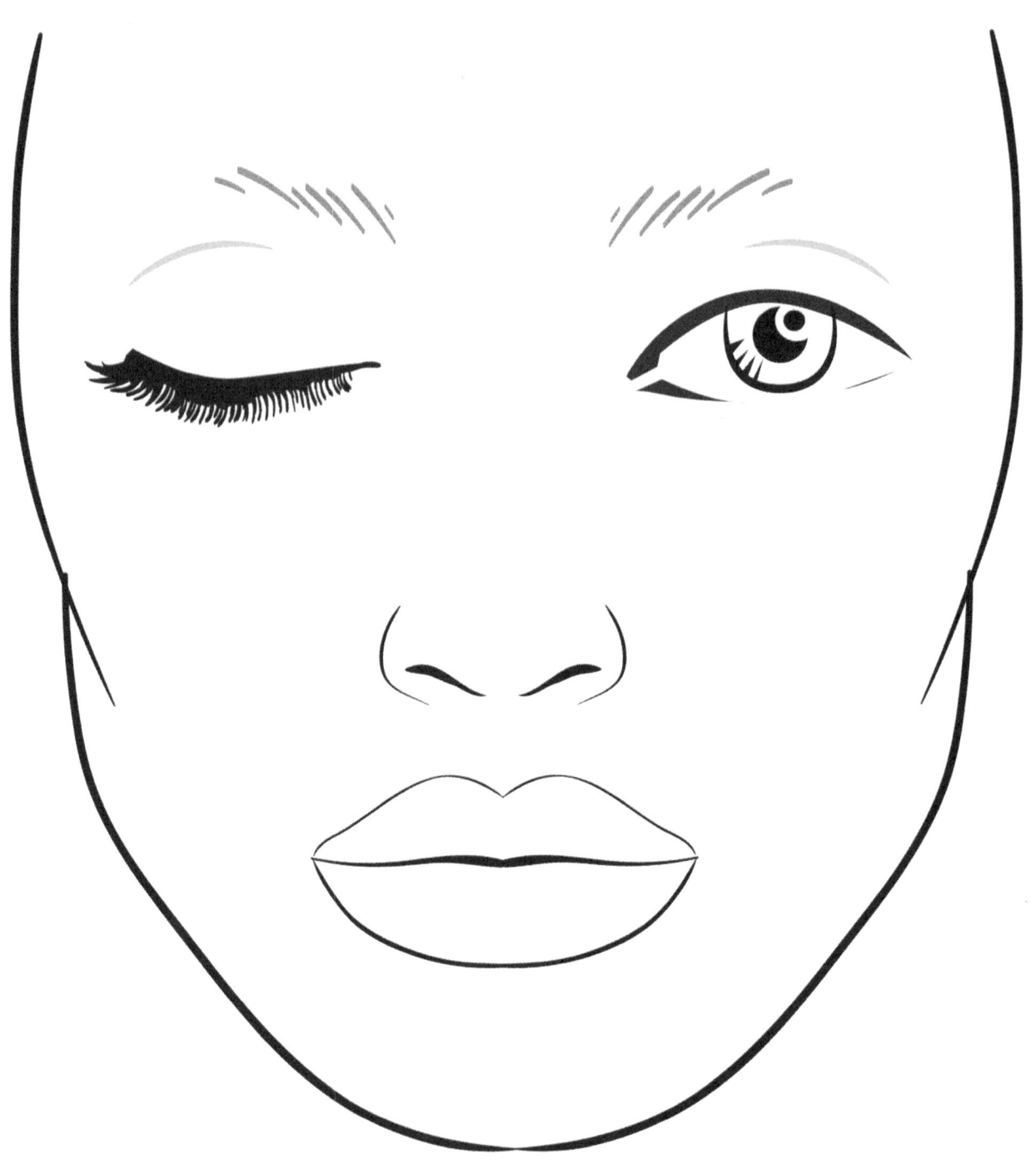

Skin	Eyes	Lips

Client Name: ....
Phone Number: ....
Email Address: ....
Makeup Look: Daytime / Evening / Wedding / Party / Other / (Circle as appropriate).

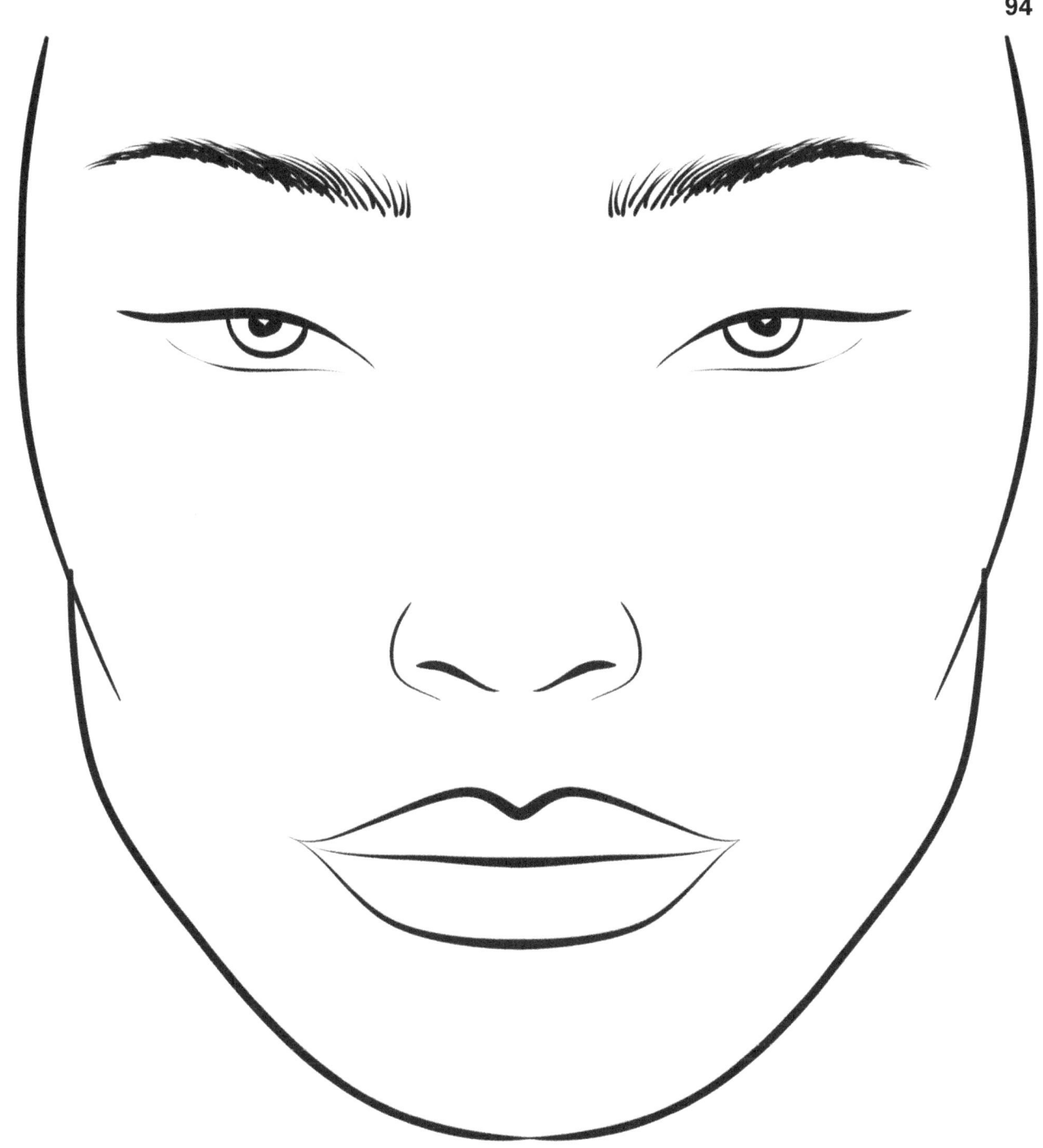

Skin	Eyes	Lips

Client Name: ....
Phone Number: ....
Email Address: ....
Makeup Look: Daytime / Evening / Wedding / Party / Other / (Circle as appropriate).

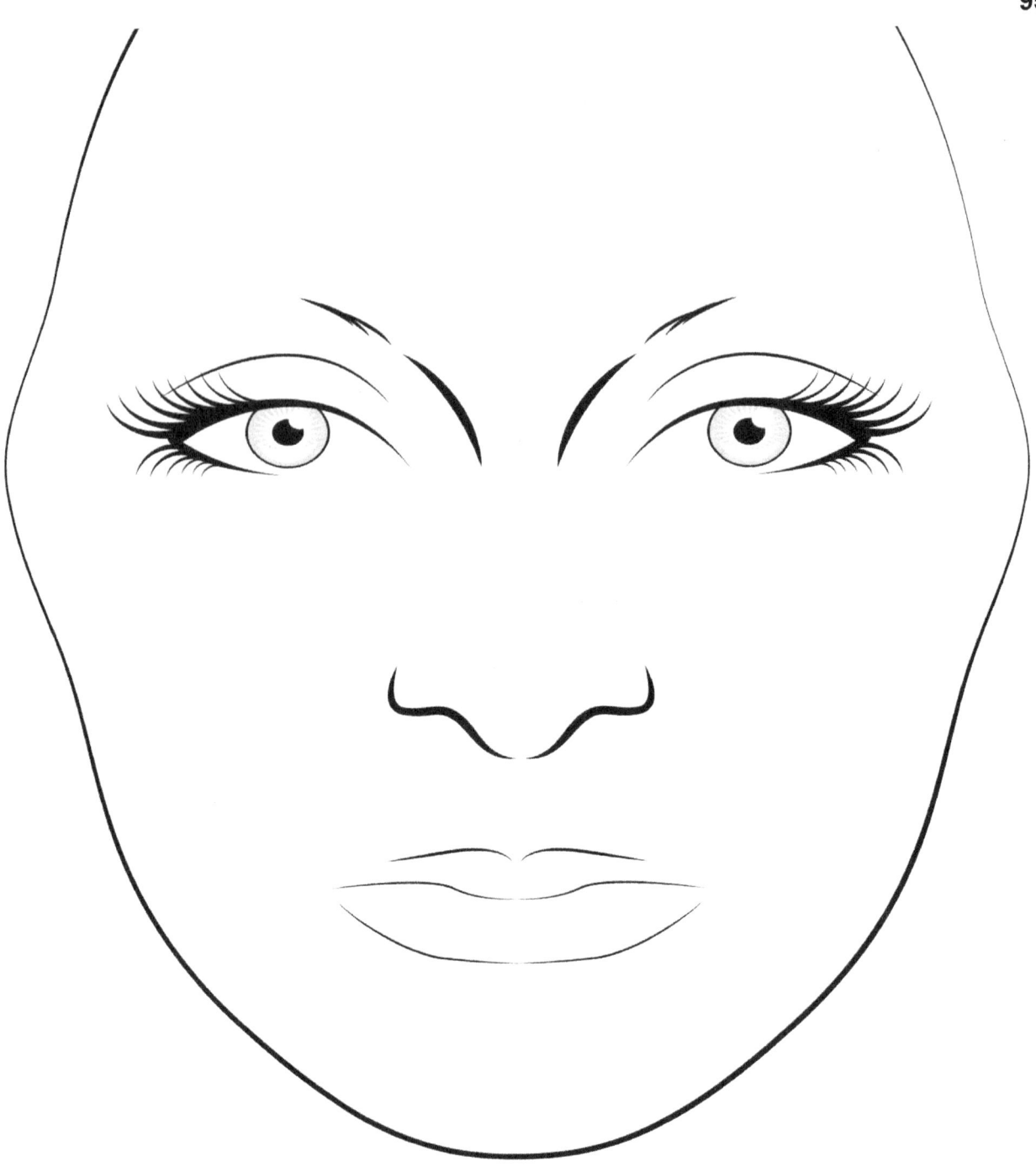

Skin	Eyes	Lips

Client Name: ....
Phone Number: ....
Email Address: ....
Makeup Look: Daytime / Evening / Wedding / Party / Other / (Circle as appropriate).

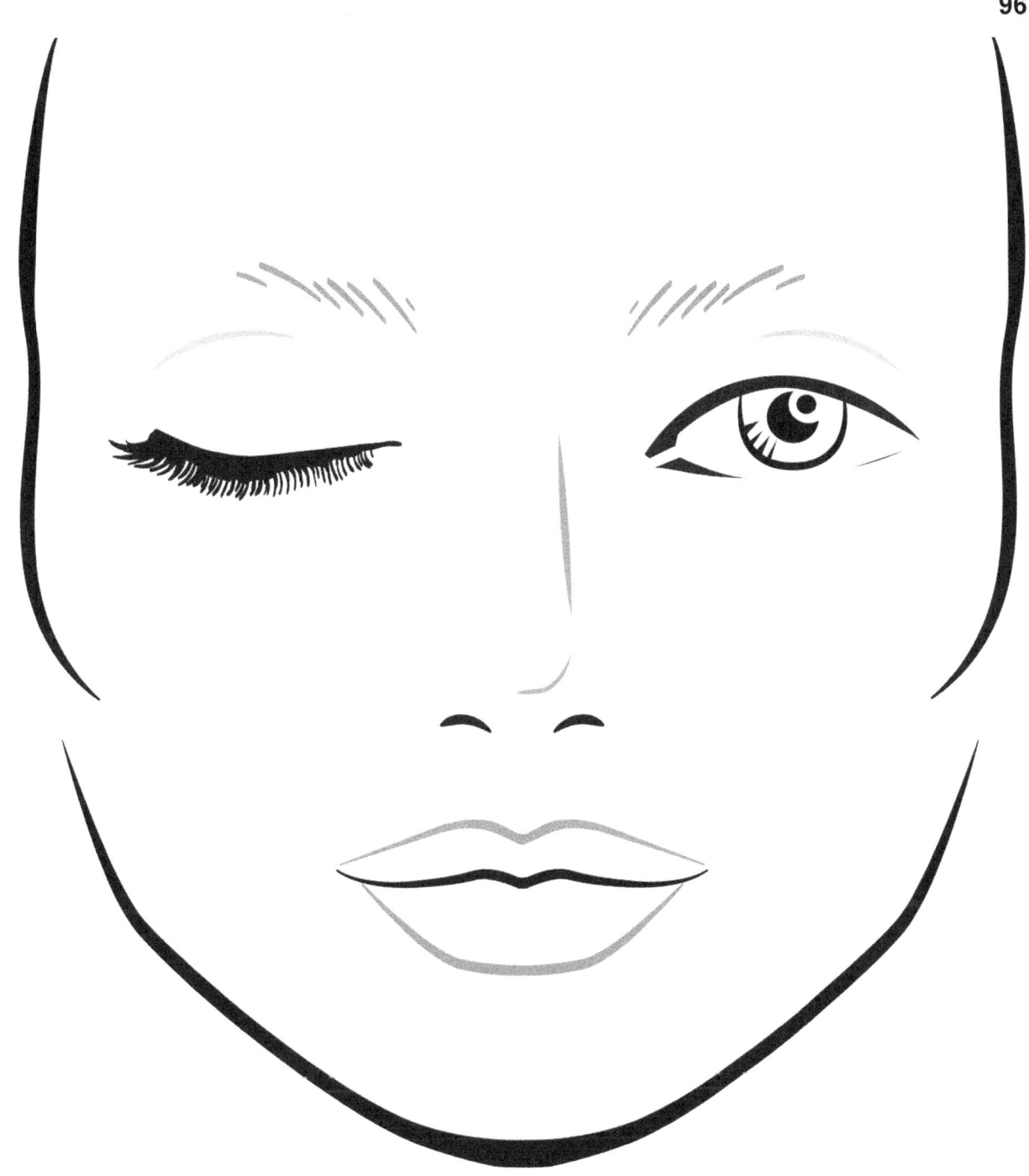

Skin	Eyes	Lips

Client Name: ....

Phone Number: ....

Email Address: ....

Makeup Look: Daytime / Evening / Wedding / Party / Other / (Circle as appropriate).

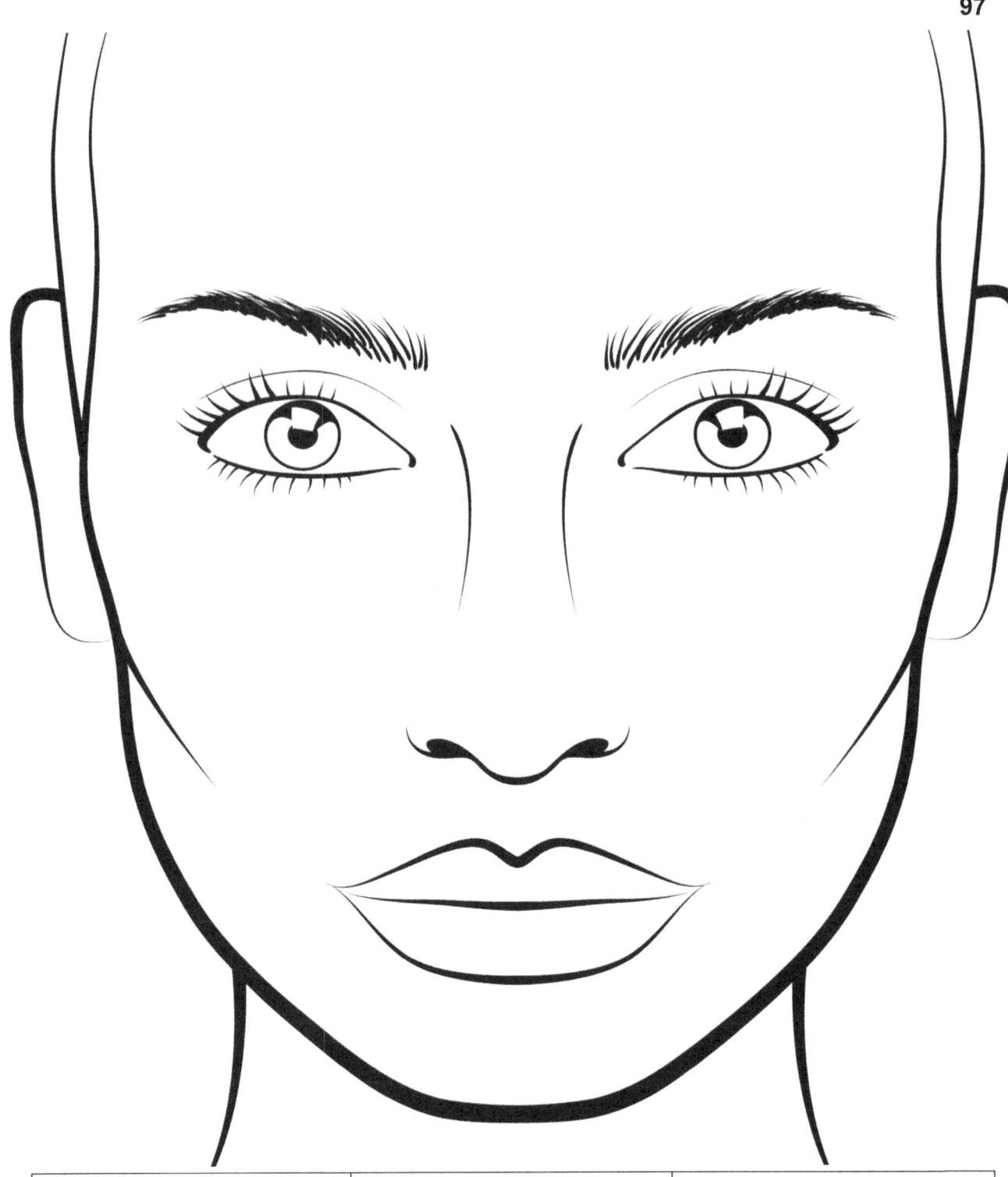

Skin	Eyes	Lips

Client Name: ....
Phone Number: ....
Email Address: ....
Makeup Look: Daytime / Evening / Wedding / Party / Other / (Circle as appropriate).

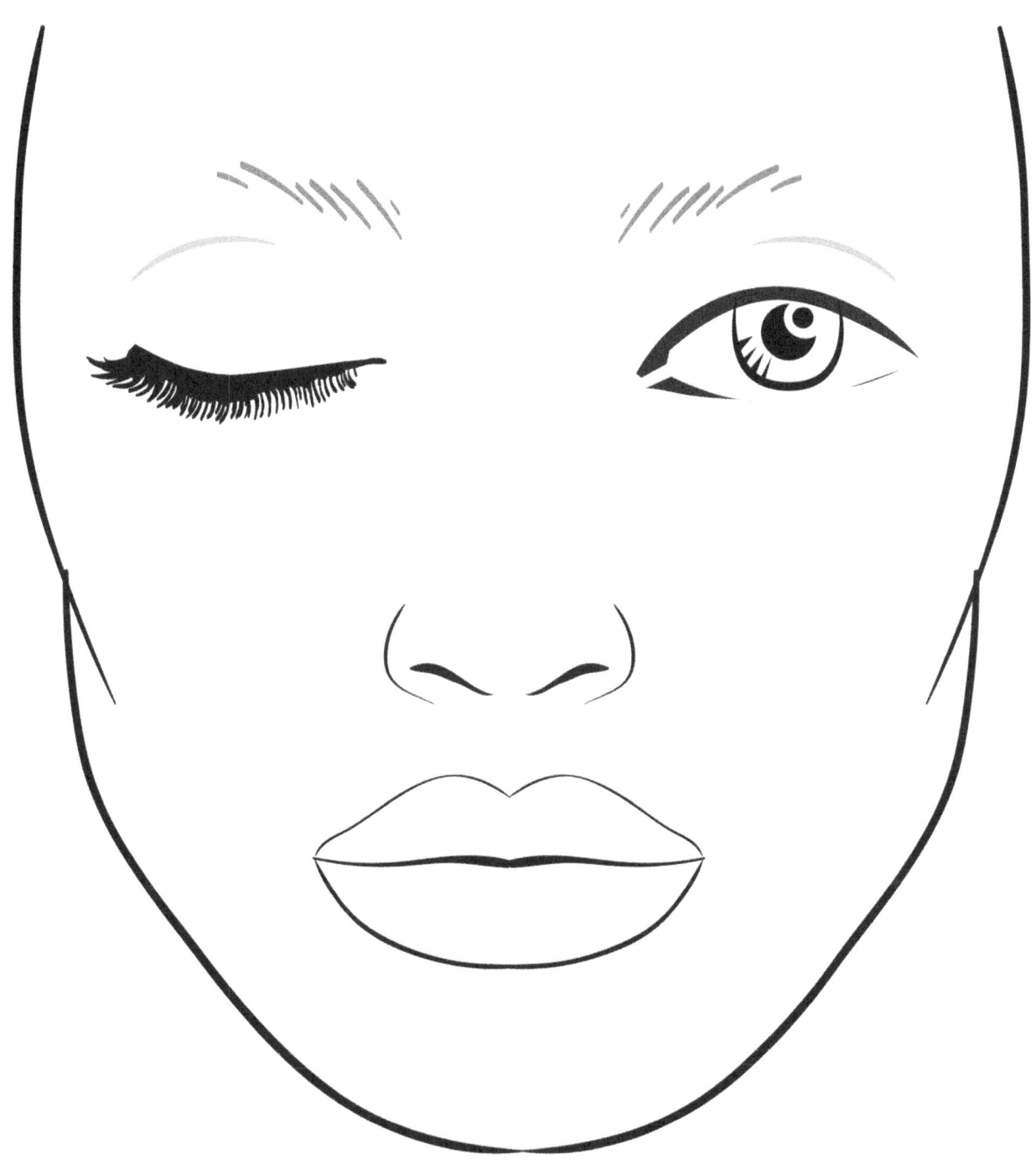

Skin	Eyes	Lips

Client Name: ....
Phone Number: ....
Email Address: ....
Makeup Look: Daytime / Evening / Wedding / Party / Other / (Circle as appropriate).

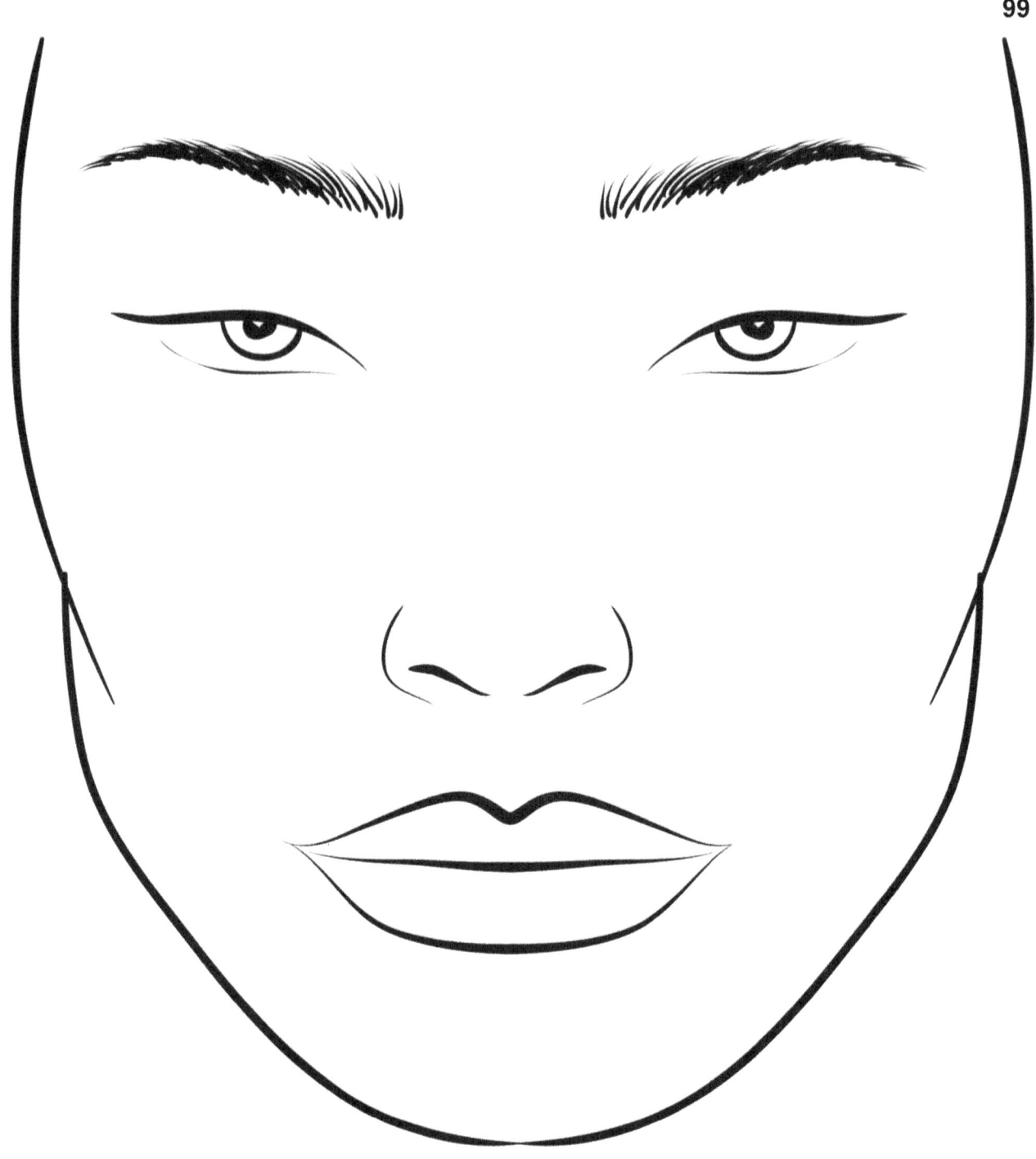

Skin	Eyes	Lips

Client Name: ....
Phone Number: ....
Email Address: ....
Makeup Look: Daytime / Evening / Wedding / Party / Other / (Circle as appropriate).

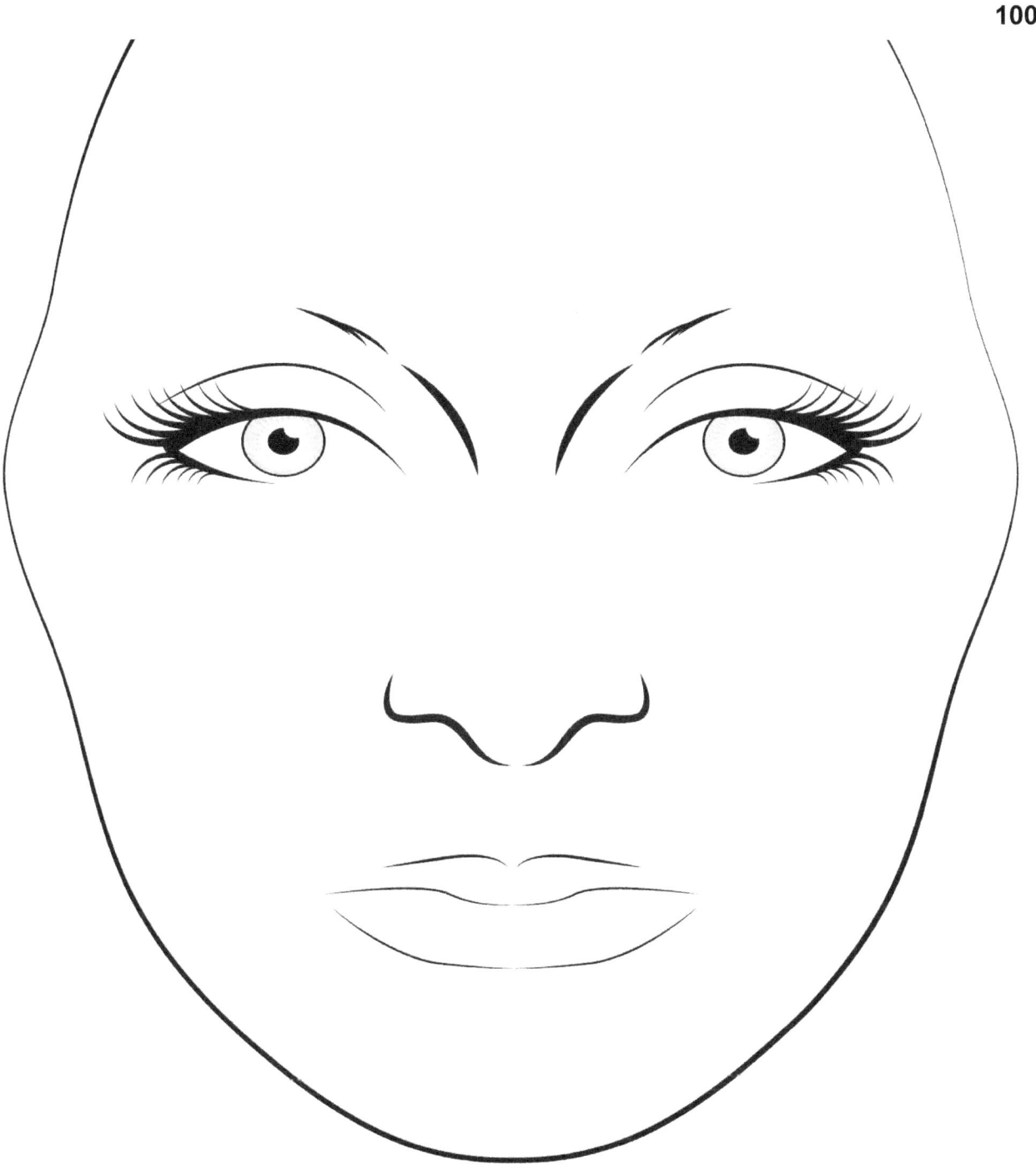

Skin	Eyes	Lips

Client Name: ....
Phone Number: ....
Email Address: ....
Makeup Look: Daytime / Evening / Wedding / Party / Other / (Circle as appropriate).

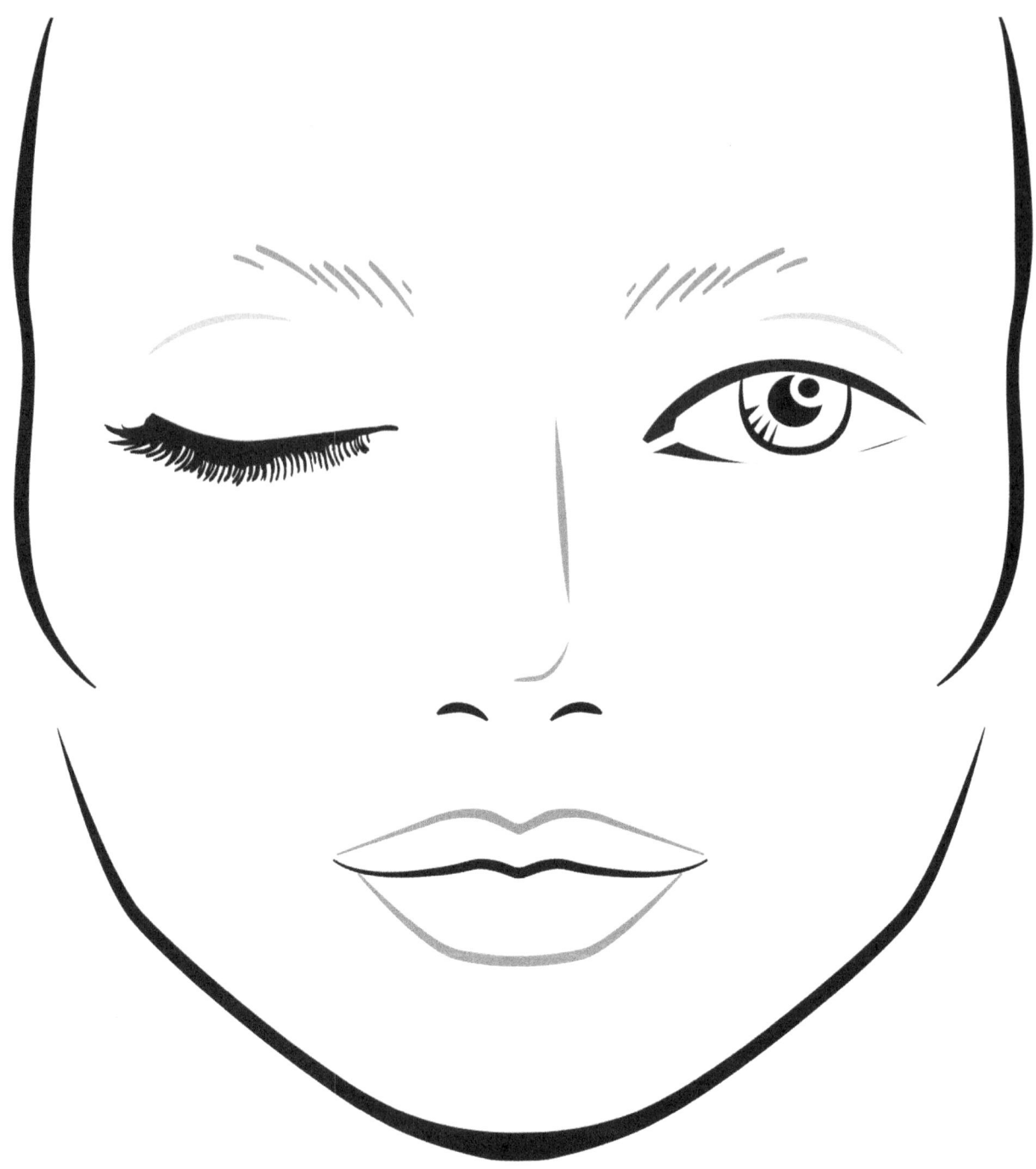

Skin	Eyes	Lips

Client Name: ....
Phone Number: ....
Email Address: ....
Makeup Look: Daytime / Evening / Wedding / Party / Other / (Circle as appropriate).